THE FAR SHORE

Let go the future,
let go the past,
let go the present,
Be on the far shore.

The Buddha
Dhammapada 318

A Word to the Reader

If you're going to spend a year alone on an island, I would recommend you take *The Far Shore* along with you. But if you are living the way most of us do, this book may be even more important for you to read. It has been so for me and still is.

Why? Because each time I read even a few lines, it has an immediate and magical effect of transporting me home to my true being. The simplicity and clarity of these words allow me to see things simply, as they are, without all the turmoil and dramas of my mind. So reading *The Far Shore* helps me remember what's real—and forget all the rest. As I return to the natural state of simply seeing—seeing what is—I am immersed in peace, nothing else matters, everything is perfect just as it is. It is then I can let go and, in a flash, I'm there—reality.

Morgana Taylor (Totnes, Devon, England)

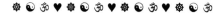

Mitchell Ginsberg (email: jinavamsa@yahoo.com), a teacher in the tradition of Buddhist Mindfulness-Insight Meditation since 1975, is the first Western disciple of Dhiravamsa, widely known and respected Thai Vipassanā Meditation Master, who as Chao Khun Sobhana Dhammasudhi formerly served as Chief Incumbent Monk (Abbot) of the Thai Buddhist Mission to Great Britain.

Since completing graduate studies in Philosophy at the University of Michigan in 1967, he has held professorships and post-doctoral fellowships at Yale, MIT, The American Institute of Buddhist Studies, UCSD (U. of Calif., San Diego), The Langley-Porter Stress Clinic of UCSF (U. of Calif., San Francisco), and elsewhere. He has been a psychotherapist and family therapist since the late 1960s.

For several years (1975 on), he led Vipassanā Meditation residential workshops in Britain, France, the United States, & Norway; since 1996, he has been moderator of the discussion group Insight Practice (a Yahoo group since 1999). He is author of "Nietzschean Psychiatry" (in Rbt. C. Solomon, ed., *Nietzsche*), "Action and Communication" (*The Human Context*, vol. VI, London, 1974), *Mind and Belief*, and *The Inner Palace*. Forthcoming are (1) *Calm, Clear, and Loving*, (2) *Peace and War and Peace, and Other Poems*, and (3) *Tango Tantras*. Full titles and more information in the end section, Books on Buddhism.

The Far Shore

Vipassanā, The Practice of Insight

MITCHELL GINSBERG

MOTILAL BANARSIDASS PUBLISHERS
PRIVATE LIMITED ● DELHI

Revised Edition: Delhi, 2009
Corrected Edition: Delhi, 2001
First Edition: Delhi, 1996

ISBN: 978-81-208-1348-9

MOTILAL BANARSIDASS

41 U.A. Bungalow Road, Jawahar Nagar, Delhi 110 007
8 Mahalaxmi Chamber, 22 Bhulabhai Desai Road, Mumbai 400 026
203 Royapettah High Road, Mylapore, Chennai 600 004
236, 9th Main III Block, Jayanagar, Bangalore 560 011
Sanas Plaza, 1302 Baji Rao Road, Pune 411 002
8 Camac Street, Kolkata 700 017
Ashok Rajpath, Patna 800 004
Chowk, Varanasi 221 001

Printed in India
By Jainendra Prakash Jain at Shri Jainendra Press,
A-45, Naraina, Phase-I, New Delhi 110 028
and Published by Narendra Prakash Jain for
Motilal Banarsidass Publishers Private Limited,
Bungalow Road, Delhi 110 007

DEDICATED TO
    the being aware
    the trying to be aware
    the being not yet ready to be aware
each of which we all have occasion to experience and learn from.

IN WARM GRATITUDE

To Dhiravamsa. To Yvonne and to Marie-Claude. To Loren and R.D. Laing. To Sam, Sylvia, Ted. To Henry, Michael, Judy. To Hans and Olga, Jacques and Orlie, Tew and Fizz, Frank and Vivian. To Manfred, Paul, Jo, Brenda, Ed. To Bob, Peter, Roland, Ann, Charles and Jean-Pierre. To Heinz Bechert and K. R. Norman. To Wendy, Hrjjayā, Fanny.
For their friendship, love, and manifesting of the dhamma.

IN ACKNOWLEDGMENT

of all who have taught and inspired me, of those who have encouraged me in the project of this book, especially of Peter, whose acute and sensitive reading of an earlier draft of *The Far Shore* has improved its flow, of Jo for the cover design and for the line drawing of the Reclining Buddha, of Paritta, Noy, and the Ven. Pra Kru Lom for the Thai calligraphy, of Jacques and Fanny for photos which they offered for use in this book, and of Dhiravamsa, Wendy, and Tew, each of whom opened the right door at the right time.

This edition, IN MEMORY of my father z"l.

CONTENTS

PREFACE

I cannot communicate by this or any other book what can only be communicated in person. Still, there is *something* I feel I can get across through writing, and I have an interest here in trying. Our communication will be greatly helped by earnest interest and a clear awareness of what I want to express to you, on my part, and an openness on your part to hear what I have to say and to see how it touches you personally.

In this book, of course, my communication to you in black and white represents living speech. I could have tried a recording instead of a book. But I have not, and so, I ask you to *listen* to what you see. If you do not hear what I am saying, I suggest that you read aloud—and see if it really doesn't talk to you.

My getting these pieces down has been easy at times, at times demanding; done sometimes in a serious mood and sometimes in a playful one, but always as a labour of love. Friends who have become acquainted with these writings these last few years tell me that they find value for themselves in them. Perhaps these pieces will touch you, too.

I find a deep poetry in clear awareness. I see that there is a power in this sort of awareness, a power to lead us to a heartfelt appreciation of life. Some might speak here of the awe we feel before what strikes us as divine or mysterious; I simply want to share some of my experience and observations with you in a way which may help you in looking at how your life is coming along and in realizing how we either move along with changing reality or work towards what we feel to be valuable in the context of life's flow. Insight here, as elsewhere, is a product of looking and so seeing.

This watchful attitude towards life was systematised long ago by the Buddha as the practice of mindfulness (sati-patthana). As this practice has as its fruit the arising of insight into life, it has also been called Vipassana (Insight Meditation).

This collection comes from various talks I have given while leading Vipassana Meditation Retreat Courses and Workshops over the past several years in England, France, and the United States, as well as from letters exchanged with friends and students. There are also a number of pages which began as part of jotted-down ideas and observations on my own. These pieces illustrate sati-patthana (open mindfulness) as the investigation into the process of consciousness.

The coming to be familiar with this *accepting* awareness, an awareness which can at the same time be very acute and crisp in its perception, occurs in many ways and is spurred on by the widest of contexts. We do not have to sit motionless in seated meditation to have this frame of mind and heart strengthen. This collection offers one such context, from the words to Ms. Kitty to the question about the mouse.

I offer this collection under the title *The Far Shore* to those of you who are on the path of self discovery and on the path of opening to relationship with others. It does not matter if you do or do not have familiarity with Buddhist Insight (Vipassana) Meditation, or with Buddhist psychology and its way of conceptualising. The far shore is certainly not limited to those who are "Buddhists".

Still, some of these writings will be especially pertinent to those who have attended vipassana meditation retreat courses and to their onflowing practice. For those of you interested in attending vipassana courses, a list of some contact addresses is given, in the section "Meditation Centres".

A few terms are occasionally used here which may not be familiar to you. A Glossary at the back gives an idea of what these various terms mean: from some possibly familiar to you such as Buddha, Dharma, Bodhisattva, and Arahat, to some lesser-known ones such as Anupassana, Sadhu, and Satipatthana.

A glance at the titles in the Table of Contents gives a feeling for the range of topics included. Some of the writings focus on issues in the practice of open mindfulness. I find that people with no background in the tradition, either practical or theoretical, follow these writings with ease. There is nothing esoteric here.

This book is not meant to be a primer in vipassana meditation, in Buddhist psychology, or in Buddhism. Following the Glossary is a list of some available books which already fulfil this function, for those of you who are interested in further study. Nevertheless, in this collection you will find Instructive Dharma, an explanation of the Dharma as the matrix of the vipassana practice, perspective, and tradition; and also, Descriptive Dharma, an illustration of Dharma as the various onflowing realities within the domain of mindfulness practice. Pieces with a manifestly Instructive Dharma aspect include "Vipassana in Munich", "Spiritual Development", "Mind Clouds", "The Past". Some of you may find this distinction unimportant. Sadhu!

Uparujjhati uddhaccaṃ
kukkuccaṃ parihīyati
cetanā cetanā yeva
ariyaṃ saccaṃ sukhaṃ mano.

Anattā khalu saṅkappā
suñño so paccayāsayo
ānāpāno va kāyamhi
annaṃ kho dhammapīti me.

อุปรุชฺฌติ   อุทธจฺจํ
กุกฺกจฺจํ   ปริหียติ
เจตนา   เจตนา   เยว
อริยํ   สจฺจํ   สุขํ   มโน

อนตฺตา   ขลุ   สงฺกปฺปา
สุญฺโญ   โส   ปจฺจยาสโย
อานาปาโน   ว   กายมฺหิ
อนฺนงฺโข   ธมฺมปีติ   เม

उपसज्झति उद्धच्चं ।
कुक्कुच्चं परिहीयति ॥
चेतना चेतना येव ।
अरियं मग्गं सुखं मनो ॥

अनत्ता खलु मङ्रप्पा ।
सुञ्ञो सोपच्चयामयो ॥
आनापानेव कायम्हि ।
अब्बखोपम्म पीतिमे ॥

Restlessness ceases
remorse is abandoned
thinking is just thinking;
truth is noble—the heart's at ease.

Plans surely have no owner
quite empty is that realm of conditioning
in the body there is breathing, in and out—
the drink of *dhamma* is indeed my nourishment.

CONVERSATION

Etadatthā kathā, etadatthā mantana, etadatthā upanisā, etadatthā sotāvadhānaṃ yad idaṃ anupādā cittassa vimokkho 'ti.

Conversation is for this purpose, consultation is for this purpose, getting close is for this purpose, listening is for this purpose — for the clinging-free liberation of the mind.

Vinaya V.164.

Sakalameva hidaṃ ānanda brahmacariyaṃ, yadidaṃ kalyāṇamittatā kalyāṇasahāyatā kalyāṇasampavaṅkatā.

Truly, the entire spiritual life, Ananda, is this — an encouraging friendship, an encouraging companionship, an encouraging intimacy.*

Samyutta-nikaya I.87-88.

To extend sincere love to one you cherish is worthwhile to each of them, the giver and receiver.

S.L.G., 25 May 1976.

*The word here, *kalyāṇa*, means beautiful, agreeable, good, noble, generous, excellent, beneficial, virtuous, auspicious, that which encourages, that which inspires; a *kalyāṇa mitta* (*mitta* means friend) — in the Theravāda Buddhist Tradition, a meditation teacher — is a good friend, a virtuous friend, a friend (in this Buddhist context) who inspires and encourages us in our process of coming to awakening and freedom.

THE FAR SHORE
(The Far Shore's Under Your Feet)

TO MS. KITTY

Petted   the cat purrs contentedly

Pushed away
by firm hand
by gruff voice   she turns away, then looks back
                       turns around and walks off
                            to the next reality
                                    easily
        letting go of unwelcoming spaces.

And you?

VIPASSANA IN MUNICH

The practice of vipassana meditation was first taught by the Buddha. It consists in the open attentiveness to what we experience. In this way we come to know and appreciate reality as it is, not as our ideas tell us it must be. Through mindfulness comes insight (vipassana).

Traditionally the practice is done in sitting, standing, and in walking postures. In our practice we go deeply into our experience, using the discipline of mindful silence to help us become more sensitive to how we in fact respond to what life actually offers us, and to be more in touch with ourselves on the physical, emotional, mental, and spiritual levels, within the limits of our conditioning, and beyond.

For sitting meditation, we have found that sitting practice with the eyes closed and for a period of about one hour allows our more profound energies to come to the surface for us to experience fully. This differs somewhat from certain other meditation traditions such as Rinzai Zen which uses eyes-open sitting for shorter periods of time.

In addition to this core of sitting practice, we also use various body-oriented exercises including free movement, dancing and perhaps shaking to music, and so forth. We are aware that various deep psychological patterns are held in the body itself, and by allowing the body to work directly with these holding or storage areas, the freeing up of these residues from the past is accelerated. (To put this into traditional terms, this is the work of burning karma.)

> For use in an announcement of a
> course to be held with the
> Munich group.

PICK ONE TECHNIQUE AND STICK TO IT

Let's not get lost in defining the word technique, and after that in determining whether vipassana meditation is a technique, BUT: What sort of attitude is being advocated when we are told to pick one technique and stick to it? And what is happening when we ourselves decide to follow one technique exclusively?

If we look, we may experience fear and reluctance: FEAR that some satisfying state we have attained might be lost, or that a direction of change we've liked might be cut off, and RELUCTANCE to go beyond what we are content with by trying something new.

All of this frequently leads to a narrowing down, a closing off, a rigidifying. This rigidifying out of fear may also lead on a grander scale to sectarianism. Have you heard these isolationist words somewhere?—

"We Mahayanists, on the other hand, . . ."
"The Adamantine Teaching, which is supreme, . . ."
"The purity of the U Ba Khin Tradition . . ."
"Those pagan heretics . . ."
"Death to all infidels . . ."

All this is simply more of what we call the net of views, the trap of views, the thicket of views, the clinging to views.

In this we see a self-limiting tendency, a defensive attitude towards, or rather *against*, an unknown future reality, a desire to keep things (onflowing reality) under our control.

We can appreciate our satisfaction, our contentment, our happiness, our joy, without freezing into immobility, without attempting to ward off change. (*Could* change be warded off?) But perhaps we *will* see such a futile attempt arise. If so, maybe we see its basis and get a perspective on it all, so that when this attempt to ward off change does ultimately fail, we are not spun into a turmoil.

At each point in the flow of life, we may see preferences being formulated for what the next moments will be like. Then we may see these preferences channelling our energies. And perhaps once in a while we will begin noticing an occasional neutrality towards the next moments: a full openness, a deep interest in what they will be, in what they are, not for what they do for us or against us, but simply because they are. This is like scientific curiosity, with heart.

ALL PATHS

All paths which lead inwards and onwards
    in tenderness and in love
Surely show their worth.

THE FAR SHORE'S UNDER YOUR FEET

We may feel some sort of "progress" or "advancement" while we are at a meditation retreat: We may have seen some difficulty for us come up, and seen it disappear. This may be followed by the idea that this difficulty will never again be experienced. That *would* be nice, wouldn't it?

So what, then, if it does arise again at some later time? Maybe you will see it on your very first day out of the retreat setting! What then?

If we let the difficulty appear again, rather than thinking it won't, and resisting it when it does, we can look further into a process that began here at the retreat, to see it end, or, if it doesn't end, to see how it continues or evolves. In either case, we let it flow through and then we are clear of it.

We can use a retreat situation as an environment where a clearing out of ourselves can take place. And we can use all of life that way; all of life can be a retreat. But it's a retreat in the world. All that is needed is the same attitude that is nurtured in a retreat setting.

This is not in the sense of having rules about how to behave: Sometimes we go to a retreat and the people there have some suggestions for us about how to act during the retreat. When we go out in the world after the retreat ends, we might think that the essence of the retreat is following certain rules.

With vipassana there is also a morality or way of right acting. Now, the way of right acting that comes from vipassana does not come through following rules. The way of right acting through vipassana is seeing what is to be done. If we are driving down the street and we see a car stop in front of us, we don't need a rule, Stop when the car in front of you stops. With insight we see that there is a car stopped in front of us. We see the right action not through a rule, but by seeing what the reality is. Appreciating the reality, we see how things are going. We act in accordance with what is appropriate to the reality. That is a kind of morality, but a morality without rules.

We don't need rules about how to retain what we have learned during this retreat, about how to keep our mindfulness from diminishing when we leave the retreat setting. To start with, though, we can already see here a desire to have something continue, which feels right to us at the present moment. Or maybe we feel a desperation about it—not merely a desire. Well then, the way we have mindfulness continue after the retreat is to continue being mindful: To keep breathing after the retreat, we just keep breathing. We don't need a rule, First there is an in-breath and then an out-breath, and we do it in that order, and continue doing it. We just keep breathing. And we just keep being mindful.

Certainly the experience outside the retreat will be different from the experience within the retreat. Even the experience within the retreat is different from the experience within the retreat: How it is now is different from how it was ten minutes ago. What you are seeing now is different from what you were seeing ten minutes ago. How your body feels now is different. So that will be the same; it will be different. It'll be different when you leave the retreat. So there may be more noise that you hear. There may be more interpersonal contact with other people. There may be more feeling of practical pressures: pressure to do this, pressure to do that.

Maybe you will be seeing a different reality. Then you will have the chance to learn more and more about yourself. By putting yourself into more and more contexts, you have a lot of lessons to learn from. We can treat reality as something that gives us problems and hassles, and something to be borne, some burden we have to carry, or some drudgery that we have to get through. Or we can treat reality as something to learn about, just to see what it is: that is mastering the mystery of Maya. Until Maya is mastered, it is reality which has the power to delude us, since we are continually misinterpreting it. Maya is mastered just by our seeing into Maya, by appreciating all the little realities that are created, all the different experiences that we come through.

We can enjoy Maya. We can understand it, and then we aren't deluded by it. We can appreciate what's happening. Then Maya is simply samsara, the on-going flow, or the circle or cycle of life. We look into samsara, appreciate it, and then it is no longer Maya for us. When we appreciate it fully—this is being in a nirvanic state, in nibbana. In Buddhist terms, we can say that samsara is nirvana.

We can talk of crossing over to the far bank. But we have to understand what the far bank is. The far bank isn't separate from samsara. The far bank is seeing through samsara so that it is no longer illusion to us, no longer Maya to us.

19

When we see all of our reality for what it is, when we allow each experience to be just what it is, without reading all sorts of interpretations into it, then we are already on the other shore. Crossing the stream of samsara is a matter of changing our experience of each moment of consciousness by allowing it to be just as it is. You don't have to travel anywhere to get to the far shore: the far shore's under your feet.

So we see beyond "this shore" and "that shore". We're in samsara but not of it: we simply experience the world of phenomena, and so we're experiencing samsara, but not being carried away by it, not being deluded by it. When we go back into "life" after a retreat, there is a chance to experience more of that, to learn more about that.

So we see if we enjoy life or if it pains us. Sometimes there will be pain. There is no guarantee that it will be painless along the way. We don't have an expectation of its being painless, or of its being painful. We just see what it is. If it's painless now, we enjoy its painlessness. But when there is pain, when there is some kind of a problem, we can look at it, we can see it. Then we can continue taking it all in stride. We don't let it build and build that way until it ends by being overpowering.

This is treating life not as a burden to be borne for a while, until death. We don't live life just waiting for death. That is not the aim of life, or the goal of life, even though it might be the end of life. We are just living and experiencing, learning, seeing what's happening, having insight, having vipassana into the way things really are, cultivating insight and growing through insight. That's vipassana living, living a "meditative" life.

SPIRITUAL DEVELOPMENT

Where are we going on this spiritual trip? Is it just more heavy luggage in a journey already replete with burdens?

Have we once again given up our ability to judge for ourselves, turning away from the problems and complications of life with some predigested "truth"?

So we're looking for something. This means we can see a dissatisfaction, an unacceptable situation, an unacceptable experience. We may feel an emptiness in the way things are, a desire to make things better, a desire to improve ourselves. And what do we imagine as a solution to this dissatisfaction?

We may look to certain people as models: We hear of someone who is so "spiritually developed" that when he sits in meditation, a light is visible glowing forth from him. Or of another who has such "spiritual powers" that a large pin stuck in a cheek causes no pain.

Are *you* that developed? And is this really the something extra you want from life? Is *this* what "higher development" is aimed at? Does *your* deepest problem come because your aura isn't the right colour?

Let's get back to earth. Here we are. Each day our time and energy flow onwards. Does it feel smooth, comfortable, acceptable? Is it sometimes rough going, painful, unacceptable? Is the flow more like a whirlpool than a brook?

If we inspect our life situation more deeply than by merely noting each separate instant of consciousness by itself, we begin to see inter-relations and patterns. Some of these involve great pain. Many show how we repeatedly resist the ongoing flow of reality, or, at least, attempt to channel it according to desires which are constantly arising.

We can appreciate this capacity to gain insight into our various ways of living in the world, and continue seeing more and more deeply how we are going through life. Or, we may find ourselves getting entangled in our *thinking* about how we are going through life; perhaps our mind will take a philosophical bent and come up with the cavalier idea that it's all illusion, all maya. But, all we need is a little deep pain to have us recover our senses.

Back with our senses, what we experience is not this or that conception of how reality *ought* to be, but the particulars of our situation as humans in this time and space. When we arise in the morning, we feel hunger in our bellies. When we feel good-willed love from others, we feel a new, special energy. When we see another in distress, we know that sadness, or wonder what it must really feel like. When we are tired, we want to rest. When our environment is beautiful, we are at peace. (Salvador Dali once said that the soul is a state of the landscape.)

The most spiritual life is the most mundane. (Put in a Buddhist way, nirvana is samsara.) The role of spiritual development is in the *active* liberation of our limited energies from all those pain-producing, self-constricting and inter-personally poisonous channels it is repeatedly flowing into.

We can get on with this liberation without becoming passive through fear of acting. And without beclouding any of our mind's natural crisp clarity.

When we truly allow every bit of reality to show itself to us, we allow in not only what we feel is good, or proper, or "spiritually developed", but anything and everything. Then we can learn from life in all it fullness. We appreciate the idea that our eyes *and* our heart will be present at *all* times (1 Kings 9: 3).

When we become open to learn from life in all its fullness, we are alive to learning more and more deeply how our lives and how our relationships in the world are coming along. We are travelling on, becoming intimately aware of how life works. This is how we carry on. "A man cannot know himself better than by attending to the feelings of his heart and to his external actions" wrote Boswell in 1762.

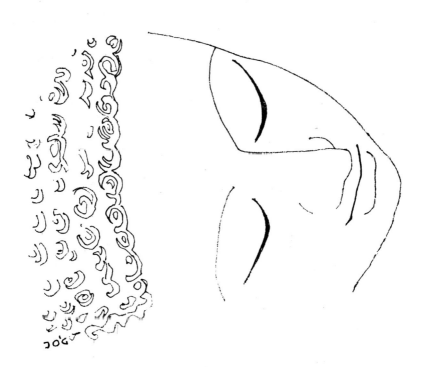

LOVE AND RESPECT

We may say that what is really important in life is love, pronounced softly and full of vibrancy in our voice, and we may feel this to be oh so true. And yet we may notice our energies going into concerns about respect.

When we look at these two, at love and at respect, it is clear that they are miles, no, worlds apart. The deep contentment and joy to be alive which are born of love just aren't generated by respect.

Respect focuses on identity, especially on socially definable identity. It has in its domain the world of credentials. I did this. I've associated with these great people. I was honoured by this significant group. I've been invited to this or that important occasion. Respect brings about comparison, evaluating personal worth, competition between people, pride and shame.

It is a losing game. Within its structure, its limits, its rules, even when we are "winning", we are only standing on the sandy ground of social fictions. We get our support from the recognition of others. And so, we lean heavily. This makes us very unstable, unsure, and ill at ease.

And, when within its structure we are "losing", we do not even have the little strength which being respected occasionally brings us by giving us some confidence. But we do have true self-disrespect: We don't like ourselves; or rather, we don't like our socially-known image. And we don't really look at ourselves (dis-re-spect: the lack of seeing ourselves).

So what, then, if we say and feel that love is what is really important in life! For, in spite of how we feel about love, we may have a deep stake in respect, in what it brings to us, especially in the initial feeling of satisfaction and superficial level of acceptance, or in its various forms of power.

The way of love is not the way of power. If we long for what the way of love involves but march down the way of power, our longings here will never be fulfilled.

We could see years if not lifetimes of frustration arising out of such a mischannelling of life's precious energies.

So it is important for us to appreciate what we experience as valuable, and what we *do*. If these are not in harmony, as when we feel the value of love and yet strive for power and distancing respect, we can look carefully to appreciate how this disharmony arises.

Perhaps we have a confusion. Maybe we equate love with respect. Recently, feeling love and friendship and goodwill for her, I hugged a seven-year-old friend of mine. She looked at me with some puzzlement and asked, What did I do that you liked, Mitchell? Perhaps in her experience, expressions of love were typically connected with approval of some form. So we may be far from the experience of love as just love, and have familiarity mostly with love for deeds done or accomplishments accomplished. Love becomes just one more form of payment to a capitalist mentality.

Such a confusion is not that uncommon. Such a confusion has powerful consequences. Such a confusion can be overcome by appreciating these consequences.

The disharmony may have other roots. When you next notice such a disharmony, what will *its* basis be? Or perhaps you will just notice, uninterruptedly, full harmony in your present life!

THE DISCOURSE ON FREEDOM THROUGH GOOD COMPANIONSHIP

My friends Michael and Judy were going to celebrate their union through a Sufi wedding ceremony, atop Mount Tamalpais. I was asked to read a Buddhist selection as part of that Universal-Worship ceremony. I looked for something not syrupy sweet, as I had the feeling that there would be enough of that without my contribution. I found an inappropriate word by Shantideva advising against relating to immature spirits (bālajana—or, fools, as some translate it), and one by D. H. Lawrence offering in a poem the idea of taking the sun from one another and leaving the valueless rest. Michael said the selection should be *obviously* Buddhist. So I put what I felt worthwhile and relevant to say to them in the form of Pali sutta. Michael asked if there was a mention of bodhisattvas and such, and so I added an uncharacteristic sprinkle of such beings among those present to hear the discourse. What came out during the ceremony, held atop Mount Tam on a beautiful April day in 1977, was this, which was given the traditional-style name of

The Discourse on Freedom through Good Companionship.

Thus have I heard. On one occasion the Blessed One was staying in the Squirrels' Grove, among the trees, and in his company were five hundred monks and five hundred lay-people, five hundred Great Beings Mahasattvas, five hundred Bodhisattvas from the ten quarters, and one thousand shining deities.

And the Blessed One saw the hearts and minds of all those in his company. And he addressed them, saying, O monks and lay-people, Mahasattvas, Bodhisattvas, deities.

And they responded, Yes O Blessed One.

And the Blessed One said, The great ocean, O friends, has but one taste, that of salt. Just so is the Great Dharma, which has but one taste, that of freedom.

And what is the *path* to that freedom, O friends? The whole of the path to that freedom, O friends, consists totally in good companionship.

To taste that freedom, O friends, walk always on the path of good companionship. Do not abandon good companionship in the hope of achieving freedom. In the Great Dharma there is no conflict between these two. Indeed, it is only in the minds of the unseeing that there appears to be a conflict here.

And what *is* this good companionship, O friends? It is careful listening to one another, it is intimacy with one another, it is helpfulness to one another, O friends. And *which* careful listening, *which* intimacy, *which* helpfulness to one another are good companionship? Those which with seeing wisdom and with heartfelt compassion are conducive to the nonclinging freedom of the heart:

These are good companionship.

Be of help, not of hindrance, O friends, to the going beyond clinging. Be of help to the going beyond fear. Be of help to the going beyond possessiveness. In this, develop the loving appreciation of one another. Indeed, this very appreciation, this love based solidly on mutual awareness, this seeing of each other's lived reality, are what lie beyond clinging. Know *this* as the path of good friendship, O friends!

And the hearts and the minds of those in the company of the Blessed One were gladdened, and they approved of the words of the Blessed One with one voice, saying, Wise and compassionate, indeed, are the words of the Blessed One.

And a great peace fell over that grove, where they all were gathered.

—Thus ends the discourse of the Blessed One entitled The Discourse on Freedom through Good Companionship (Kalyāṇamitta-tāvimuttisutta).

THE FLOWER

The flower
>   wide-open to the warming sun
Shuts up tight
>   against the cold-night wind.

Karuna-pati asks: Is one less beautiful than the other?

The Commentary says at this point, the flower is our tender heart.

YOUR ANGER

Your anger slashes thorugh me, sabre-sharp.
I cry for the two of us.

Remembrance of warmth leads to hopes of a rebirth and a rekindling
of those now-gone, once-harmonized feelings. Here, hope is a fish-
hook in our heart!

I SEE NO LIMITS

I see no limits to this pain I feel.
This love is one with the hurt
                          pain
                          torment.
Sad is this growing separate
when once there was oneness.
I see you clearly
with love that breathes through all
          my body
I cannot remove you from
even one cell of my being.
Else, I am empty.
So many tears.
In the end, a soft quiet.
Gentle slow breaths.

29

ACTIVE PATIENCE

the pain
the looking away
the slip into oblivion

the dark pit
the lost soul
the helplessness

the giving up
the letting go

the sense of clouds, of fog
the sense of time
the sense of limit

the sense of end
the sense of direction

the will to look

the joy of change

the strength to look
the sight of progress

the energy to flow

the harmony
the nonresistance
the welcoming

the unlocking
the floating
the freedom.

MAKING WAR ON EGO

There is so much hostility! We talk of "choiceless awareness", attentiveness to experience which is non-judgmentally open to any and whatever mental-physical occurrence. But we still experience dis-pleasures, dis-satisfactions, frustrations.

Perhaps our awareness is keen at these moments. Experience may perceive patterns, in which these frustrations precede later attacks, criticisms, or angry outbursts (in bodily action, word or in thought/imagination). As is said, frustration leads to aggression. What happens may be noticed when the frustration-aggression involves us and others, or simply us and ourselves.

Our painful patterns may lead to a desire to have them end (a form of the thirst for extinction, vibhava-tanhā, spoken of in Buddhist psychology). This sometimes takes the form of a resolution: I won't criticise again. Or as a wish: I wish these petty ego activities were fully stopped. Iconography represents this ego-stoppage by a large central figure holding down a tiny, struggling person by stepping on it firmly.

This is making war on ego. Besides being a manifestation of dualistic thinking, or alienated experience, it nurtures resistance to our process. Rather than learn from the situation, how we ("ego") are functioning, we reject the process and attempt to annihilate or at least fully suppress it.

A resolution often darkens our clarity of perception, so that we do not see the dis-satisfying mechanics. When we cannot see in sufficient detail to dismantle the damaging contraption, we waste energy in our overkill activity: rather than loosening one screw, we try to pulverise steel! So we must be aware of the feeling of resolution which often accompanies the making of a resolution. This is blindness pretending to be perspicacity.

But seeing into the process is difficult when we are militant against it. Hey! Are you still doing that horrible thing!

31

Now, what kind of a response will *that* bring about? An open, caring curiosity and love about the "horrible thing", or a self-defensive, strongly identifying with the thing as one's own action? Say! Now *that's* worth looking into more! That's important! It can be very freeing to understand how that works better, how each step of that process moves into the next!

We can relate to frustrating patterns in ourselves and in others with either of these two attitudes.

Welcoming in these processes, as opportunities to see what was unseen, to understand what was not understood or was misunderstood, to be clearly aware of what was not in awareness—this welcoming frees our energies for the function of investigation rather than channelling them into suppressing these processes.

The Buddha did not attempt to kill Māra. He simply saw what Māra, the friend of the deadened, the death-like, was up to. He saw Māra's attempts to distract from awareness. And then Māra was powerless. All this without hostility: Hello, Māra! What are you doing *now*? Oh, I see.

And then Māra would go away.

Anyway, that's the Buddha and Māra.

With us, maybe we'll see our ego, our desires for love, and security, and self-aggrandisement, and respect, in play (friendly or hostile) with another ego. If we are hostile to these processes of ourselves, we can see that hostility ooze over to the similar processes of the other. And vice-versa. This hostility may arise from earlier frustrations. When we can see all this, we're not tied into it: at first not so deeply; gradually, not at all.

When we see these processes occurring, we can learn compassion, be compassionate. This ego is a needy thing, but it is ignorant about what it wants, and is destined to be frustrated (in part because of this ignorance). The ego is self-frustrating, like a drop of water which rests on the shore and longs to know the sea, not realising that it is not held back from entering the sea and becoming one with it. Poor ego! Can we give it love and our sympathy (but not condescending pity)? Or do we demand of ego, a non-egoic "enlightened" perspective? Isn't that a silly thing to expect from ego? Why, then, later attack *it* for not fulfilling *our* silly demands?

32

WE WANT NOT TO SEE

We want not to see what we take to be painful or ugly.
So we don't look.
From not looking comes not seeing.
From not seeing comes not knowing.
From not knowing comes lack of confidence.
From lack of confidence come vulnerability, brittleness, fragility.
From vulnerability and such comes fear.
From fear comes defensiveness.
From defensiveness comes hostility.
From hostility comes lack of understanding of others.
From lack of understanding comes lack of compassion.
From lack of compassion comes superficiality of relationship.
From superficiality of relationship comes frustration in the sphere of love.
From love frustration comes pain.
Not wanting to see pain or ugliness, we close ourselves in, creating some of the very pain we will later have to experience or avoid experiencing.
When see this is the price we pay for not looking, we are more willing to look even at what we take at first glance to be painful.

POSING DILEMMAS

We are in the middle of something. Some activity is ongoing. The question arises, What should I do here? We may see an urge to go on with what is happening and at the same time a contrary urge to cut it off: Should I keep on with this, or am I off course, off the Middle Path, and should I change course?

Here we are posing a dilemma to ourselves. Here we feel a decision may be appropriate. Do we stick ourselves on one of the two horns of our dilemma and call that a decision, a solution? Let's not forget: There is no decision that has to be made. First, we either notice and appreciate that a dilemma is being posed, or, we do not. Then, we perhaps see that this is arising out of a conflict that we feel, no longer sure and content within ourselves about what is happening, about what we are doing, or, we do not.

If patience is allowing us to stay with this situation, if we do not attempt to "resolve" this situation by taking a stand on what ought to be done, then we will have the opportunity to see what our uneasiness is about, to see what is underlying those questions which arose a moment earlier.

Since there is some sort of conflict here, we will see more than one thing here: there will be here at least two unharmonious elements, such as interests, desires, concerns, and perhaps several or even many. And perhaps we will appreciate what is disturbing us on several levels—specific desires, general attitudes, even life plans of ours coming in here.

In this investigation (anupassanā) we have left behind looking at ourselves as simple, unified beings: "That bothers me because I am who I am."

Now, we see more clearly the various elements which make us up: What we see are particular desires, preferences, feelings, hopes, fears, images, thoughts, whatever. Here we see, in Buddhist terms, the dharmas which we note, in sequence, when we practice mindfulness. We shift here to seeing these various discreet factors of consciousness, discreet yet clearly interrelated, inter-influencing. And now, whether we *use* the language of "I" and "mine" and "you" and "yours", or not, we are in a position to appreciate these various and distinct active tendencies within ourselves which are structuring our joys and sadnesses.

One function of the oft-repeated Zenny questions such as "Who is the 'I' who desires?" and "Who is the 'I' who sees?" and so forth, is to bring about this shift.

But perhaps we do see a decision coming up, and we feel that the issue *has* been resolved. The tension we felt while stuck between alternatives feels relieved. We can relax.

We know from experience that deciding after deliberating relaxes us. It definitely has an immediate calming effect. This effect may only last a moment before the nagging question arises of whether our decision was the proper one, but a short-lived effect is as real as an enduring one. Yet, here we remember that decisions only push our energies in one of the two or more directions involved, but do not eliminate the unharmonious elements which a moment before were all active in our minds (and bodies). In this way we see more clearly that disparate desires and so forth are not harmonised by a decision, but some merely redirected, some suppressed, some nurtured, etc.

The attitude of mindfulness is one of What is going on here?, of What are the roots or sources of these vacillations and deliberations?, and not one of What should I decide here?

NUTS

Why can't we eat just one salted nut and stop?

Well, we can.

If we stop after just one, we notice that the taste lingers on. This taste brings back to mind what we have just eaten. It has us be conscious of our recent mouth-centred experience. The taste fades slowly and various images and ideas and thoughts about it come and go. This experience is subtle; it is *enough*—*if* we allow it to evolve just as it *is* evolving.

This subtle experience can bring on a reaction in the mind. The mind often prefers strong experience to subtle experience, as when it, going dull on a monotonous ache, longs for sharp pain. It becomes impatient, as if being tickled too lightly.

Here we see the mind hesitating at letting our experience be and simply becoming more alert if what is happening is not "loud" enough. We see, instead, its tendency to intensify, to amplify the experience somehow.

This interferes with the process and *its* own natural speed (slowness) and intensity (blandness). Then, whether the process is that of the fading taste of a salted nut or of any occurrence in our life, we don't experience such a process according to *its* own rhythm, but, rather, according to how *we* feel most comfortable.

Then we frequently find the desire to have the process grow "louder" (tickling anxiety). Or, the desire for it to have disappeared and ended already (loss anxiety). Either such desire tends to cut off our simply *watching* a process dissolve on its own, following its own nature.

Can we see how often we go in a karmic way here, in general?

EMPTINESS FOR THE DISTRACTED MIND

Sometimes we feel totally distracted. There's just no concentration. We are tossed all over the place, so that we are lost. We have lost ourselves.

This is almost right, almost correct. But we have a body, and so our energy is never totally scattered. We can't get *totally* spaced out.

The body is there (here) when we feel distracted. If we feel distracted, first we recognise the distracted mind. If we are lost we can look for ourselves. And if we can look we will always find ourselves; the body is something we always have with us. So we look and see: "Oh, here we are."

We can stay with the body when we feel a lack of concentration. Not in the way of blocking out from our awareness what might be distracting us, but as the centre from which we experience. When sounds come to us, we hear them. We do not have to go out to them. We stay at our centre, and let all of our experiences come through us. This centre is nothing special, nothing particular. In itself it is nothing, only the possibility of experience, only the place of emptiness in which experiences can happen. We let sounds in. They can go in one ear and out the other. We do not try to hold them in our head. We simply notice them fully as they come through our centre. Then when they are done, they are gone.

So we do not have to reach out for experience. We are fully open, letting in, and then out, all experience. We stay resting, fully in touch with the flow, and totally without being swept away and drowned by it all. We are like the tortoise. It pulls in all its limbs, its head, its tail, reaching out to nothing. But it is not disconnected, dissociated from its environment. It is still in the context it's in. It still has contact. But it is not grabby; it does not lose stability by over-reaching. We allow ourselves body-awareness, we stay aware of our body, and we too stay undistracted, knowing where we are, what we feel, open to all experiences flowing through us.

MIND CLOUDS

When we sit down in a quiet place and begin to notice the flow of consciousness, its initial noisiness becomes evident to us. Rather than experiencing calm tranquillity, we see before us a mind like a butterfly. It darts unpredictably all over our field of consciousness, landing for an instant now here, now there, and then it's off again. If we try to catch hold of this butterfly-mind it can become strongly elusive.

Our reaching out for this darting-about mind can be frustrating, tiring, and discouraging. We feel we are having a bad meditation and then we wonder if we will ever do the thing correctly. It didn't *sound* so difficult, after all, this simply being watchful!

At such times the noisiness of the mind may become drone-like, hypnotic. Awareness is out of focus. We feel ourselves in a psychological fog. We know the mind is not still, we know something is happening, but we cannot notice what it is. Experience may be very smooth and in a way even peaceful, like being enveloped in a cocoon or in a billowy cloud. We float along with little agitation. Perhaps it becomes so smooth that we hunch over or even tilt over. Our head may drop as we fall asleep, perhaps we catch ourselves snoring. Snoring is a way we have of waking ourselves up.

We realise we are floating along not noticing very clearly what is going through consciousness. Long memories or contemplations of some future situation or even sheer fantasies make up the contents of our day-dreaming. And our later recollection of our day-dreams is very selective. When we snap out of a day-dream we can return to perhaps one or two scenes from the dream. That is the limit of our awareness.

There are even times when we are totally oblivious to what is happening, even to the feeling that we are missing something. Obliviousness is totally forgetting an experience from the instant it occurs onwards. And when we are totally unaware of what is happening we are like the walking dead. Is death what we want from life?

If we are sitting with the intention of practising mindfulness, and this is what our flow of consciousness is like, great discouragement and doubt may come up. When this happens we *use* this energy which is initially "negative". We welcome it. When we make no attempt to suppress this negative energy, we do not exhaust ourselves. Instead of resisting the doubt and the discouragement, we guide their flow by our attentiveness to them. In this way *they* become polite guests and *we* are not controlled by their "negativity". Instead they provide us with energy which we use in a way helpful to our meditation. So this doubt and discouragement can be changed from powerful enemies to useful allies: Our lack of clarity is likened by the Buddha to a fire which is burning low. And what is needed to bring the fire to a healthy state again is dry kindlingwood, which is whatever helps by energising the psychological process. Doubt and discouragement make excellent kindling wood!

We may first notice the old rut of our going along here criticising ourselves, depressing ourselves with our ideas of what we conceive a good period of meditation to be. This rut may seem hard to get out of. But when we let go of the ideas of good meditation and bad meditation, we can more easily get on with the meditating, which is to say, on with simply noticing whatever comes into awareness, its origin, its growth and development, and its deterioration and ending. We watch the full life of these objects of awareness, and then we understand them. And this is no different from our understanding ourselves.

So perhaps we are feeling that we are stuck in the cloud-like state of mind, and we begin experiencing discouragement and doubt. How do we treat this experience? We notice its presence. We see what the discouragement is, what the doubt is. We do this by investigating how each of these appears to us. Then we see that each such appearance is simply one more object for awareness.

The mind may suggest that we are stuck just too strongly here to get unstuck. The thought may occur to us that this sleep-like state of mind has its own onrolling momentum, difficult to slow down or to stop. This thought is a theory. An idea about what is and what isn't easy. But we can fully acknowledge this idea. We see just how difficult it claims the task is, really see what this theory is claiming, and then we check it out, like sceptical but open-minded scientists in search of the truth.

We can see that energy is available from this self-discouraging and doubting. Of course *their* aim is to discourage and to keep us from carrying on in the practice. That is O.K. What else would we expect self-discouraging and doubting to be aimed towards? But there is no need to go where they lead. So we acknowledge them asking What are you up to now? What are you designed to discourage? What is to be doubted?

It is important to look at these new arrivals. We must learn what has brought them about. We see what they are to do, how the discouraging and the doubting are *supposed* to function. And then they are powerless.

Or does it all still feel hopeless? Do you have the idea of giving it all up at such a point? Concluding that there's nothing really to be gotten from something as silly as simply sitting, motionless! And you *know* it's not comfortable! Perhaps the thought comes, I think I'll have a smoke or a drink, or some company, some loving, or read a book, dance or listen to some music. And on and on.

So what is the reality here? There is surely quite a bit here to notice. Investigation now will be quite fruitful, energising. And this is exactly what is needed for our fires which had burned down. So we look at just this point in time: Our awareness was still low, nothing was yet especially clear. So what was in our consciousness was out of focus. We couldn't quite make it out. This is the first thing we acknowledge.

Have you ever felt that you *almost* see something just before you again sink into one more period of obliviousness? We can shift now when such a feeling arises again into looking at the lack of focus. We look at how it's working.

When something is out of focus, what *is* happening? We can imagine focusing our vision at some point. If an object is not at this focal point, it will be out of focus. When in meditation things are out of focus, are *they* not at the focal point, not at the right place to be seen clearly? But how can they *not* be at the right place? After all, what is being looked at *here*, in meditation, is what is happening in consciousness, is what is the present-ed, present reality. And reality is *always* at the right place. Surely if we want to see the present reality, we have to look where *it* is, not where we want or imagine it to be.

So we have something here influencing our gaze. Our gaze is not focused on what's happening. So why is what is happening out of focus? If we are looking out of focus we can change our focus. Perhaps we have been trying to perceive an impressionist painting with an electron microscope. Surely we can put down the microscope, then.

But how do we know how to look, where to look? This is no question. We do not have a problem here, only our desire to have

40

it all set up for us beforehand with a money-back guarantee. But we're in the wrong show-room for that! Reality writes no guarantees.

So why *don't* we have a problem? Because we do not need to know where to look, how to look. We just look. We must give up the idea that we know where to look and then we will be able just to look: We see what is most easy to see. For that's what there is to look at. If mindfulness meditation has any rule, it's simply, *Notice whatever is most prominent in consciousness and continue on doing that.* That's all. If it's getting hard, just look again. Perhaps you will notice then that you are unnecessarily straining. Now, do you see what leads to that straining?

Perhaps in your desire to get out of this mental torpor you have focused on the breathing sensations. Then when this fails, you may remember that the Buddha looked at this, looked at concentrating when there is low awareness. And he compared it to someone's responding to a low fire trying to revive it by heaping on wet leaves.

So you may work at finely focusing the attention on the breath at the tip of the nose, or on the movements of the belly in breathing, until all awareness is overcome by sleepiness, all yawning is gone, and sound sleep takes over. If we are too finely focused we will be as good as blind. If our full body is all which we can barely perceive, can we accept that as the object of meditation? If not, we are blinding ourselves here with a rule about what is or isn't an appropriate meditation object.

It is important to look at this preference for one meditation object over another whenever we come across this mental drowsiness, known in Buddhism as Sloth and Torpor, the Third Hindrance. Can we see what our preference in the given instance is? Something *is* arising in consciousness which we prefer *wouldn't* be. Or something is *not* arising in consciousness which we prefer *would* be. So we are separating ourselves from whatever the present reality is. We are separating ourselves from reality, keeping ourselves back, and this is known in Buddhism as dukkha, and known to all of us as living reluctantly through a dissatisfying experience.

Can we see this dissatisfaction clearly? Can we look into what preferences are alive here? Can we see these preferences bringing about our resistance to what is happening, to the present stage of ever-changing reality? Why are we working so hard to make difficulties for ourselves? We can see, each of us, what in this and what

41

in that context is disturbing to us, what we do to resist, and what brings on this resisting. When we see the harm we do to ourselves out of ignorance and lack of skill in our activities, we learn skilfulness, practical wisdom. Then there can be an end of these activities which we found harmful. The way out of the pain of carrying something burdensome is to lay down the burden. It is the stopping of *all* such practices which we call nirvana. But what follows is not the end of *everything*; what follows is simply the end of the pain those practices entail.

There is in every unclear mind some preference for reality to be other than it is. What do we want not to be happening? If we ask ourselves this question, and then do *not* attempt to figure out the answer, but rather simply let come whatever comes to mind, we will be approached by the answer. All that is helpful for us is to be waiting patiently and attentively.

But perhaps when we pose this question, and let the answer come, it will be painful for us. It might even be the very dissatisfaction which is at the root of our present unclear, foggy, or wandering mind. So. Is this in turn just an idea, a premonition, a fear we use to keep from seeing the reality which we enslave ourselves by? We see this idea, this fear, but we still look to see what comes to us: We look at the reality long enough to see our reactions, to learn what biases and inclinations there are still alive in us. Slowly we become free of them through this seeing. *This path to freedom is a gradual path.*

When we pose this question about our preferences, do we painfully glimpse that root dissatisfaction once again? *Did* we get a glimpse of it once again just then? Is it back in all its original painfulness? Does this reopen an old wound?

Do we have a painful old wound here? If so, we can see now that this wound which still pains us has never been properly cared for. Here is our chance. Now we can finally treat our wounds successfully. So what is there for us doctors to do? When we were little children we used to play doctor. All we had to do then was to bandage imagined cuts over. We do not have to limit our helpful procedures *now* to what we then played around with. Our insight has certainly grown since *then*! We must learn now how to help our wounds heal. We can be grateful that these wounds of ours are so patient that they will reopen for us over and over while we try different treatments, until we learn how to heal! Why chase away, then, our best teachers? We look now. We carefully examine what needs treatment, and then we *see* the treatment which is appropriate. Or do we really think, even now, that, no matter what the wound, a big enough bandaging will not only *cover* but *heal* it?

So it is time to look. We look here without knowing what we will see. We do not even know if we will be experiencing a wound, a foggy or a clear consciousness. Our *thought* that we have mental drowsiness, and our dissatisfaction about this drowsiness could combine to convince us that we know our state of mind. But this I-know-how-I'm-feeling attitude will blind us to clarity of awareness as it emerges. So *we keep a check that this attitude does not take control.* Then we may notice, Oh, everything is quite clear again! Or perhaps what is most striking in our consciousness is the intensity of the reopened wound, the present dissatisfaction. Pain whether physical or psychological has the capacity to bring about impressive clarity!

So we note well this present dissatisfaction. No one said that it would be comfortable for us to look at what is making us uncomfortable. But it is uncomfortable for us either way. Yet, if we bring deep attentiveness with us we can let go of everything else, everything painful, and so get through the troubled waters we occasionally meet in life's journeying. Do we have the patience and the courage to help ourselves through these? With mindfulness, the waters we go across are more invigorating and enjoyable than we sometimes suppose them to be.

There is true living waiting for us if we are continually watchful: With this mindfulness we can end our death-like state and fully *live* through life's journeying. We call this, voyaging over to the far shore.

THE DESIRE FOR FREEDOM

Life brings with it not only pleasures but also pains. We can see this, and when this is clear to us, when we have no doubt about this, we may see a desire arise to be free of this pain. This is a desire for freedom.

We can want freedom. We can see how this desire for freedom works and also, maybe, how it is kept from working.

Sometimes we take on a theory about desires and how they are *all* undesirable, how *any* desire is tied in with pain, and so it doesn't matter what the particular desire is; any desire is a desire and to be avoided.

This idea can lead us to fight the desire for freedom, to resist it. If we *look* at desires, we *can* see that every desire *is* a desire. We can also see that certain desires lead in one direction, and other desires lead in another direction. There's a difference here between different desires, even if they are all alike in one way. There is the special desire, to end all desires. If we cut against that desire, if we suppress that desire and its force, there is not the energy to break away from the systems we are locked into, from the conditioning that we are.

We have a conditioned aspect to ourselves. This wants freedom, too. Freedom sounds nice. "Yes, I would like to be free." Attracted toward this freedom, we think, "Oh, I'm going to a two-week meditation retreat. I hope I'll leave it enlightened. *That's* all I really want! "

This desire for freedom is coming from conditioning. We can see here how conditioning imagines freedom to be: a state in which the conditioning has its own way, where the desires coming out of conditioning run rampant, unrestrictedly. That's called freedom of the self, freedom of the ego. This is like being released from prison: the end of external constraints on self-fulfilment.

Freedom *of* the self is freedom for conditioning to form deeper and deeper ruts, working towards its preconception of what will satisfy.

Freedom of another sort is freedom *from* the self, freedom from the ego, from the conditioned mind, freedom from conditioning.

Out of this very conditioning, out of this conditioned mind, comes an "understanding" of freedom, which is a limited understanding of freedom. It must be limited: like a fish which has no experience of the dry land, no basis for knowing what is beyond the lake it knows as its world. Its limit is its lake; its lake is its conditioning.

Still, conditioned mind tries to go beyond the conditioning, and even wants to be that which goes beyond the conditioning. But of course conditioned mind, the conditioning, cannot go beyond conditioning.

We simply let this conditioning be, as limited as it is. We do not stay in its confined world by arguing with it, or fighting it. To go outside we don't destroy the building we're in; we just go outside. And where is this outside? It is not literally somewhere else!

In moving along the path to freedom, we do not have to direct ourselves in any given direction, or go anywhere at all! In fact, when we notice a channelling of the flow of life, we can see the work of our preconceptions, of our limited desires, of one or another aspect of our conditioning. There is nothing "wrong" or "bad" about this. But we are not deluded into thinking that this is something it isn't. It isn't seeing into conditioning and its manifestation; it *is* that conditioning and manifestation. All there is to do is to appreciate how this conditioning can work at very subtle or very sublime levels. We know that when this is not clearly appreciated, there is often a tendency for pride to arise, a possessiveness about what is imagined to be a very "high" state! This is just one more form of creating a self-image.

We can watch here how our preconceptions, or, to use a word, how the ego, tries to regulate the flow of life. We watch how it doesn't know where to go, but thinks that it knows. We can watch how it usually steers away from pain.

We can see how strong this tendency to avoid pain is in us; it's a very strong tendency. It's much easier, or, rather, sometimes it *feels* much easier, to get into loving and joyful feelings. It's very difficult then to feel the negativity that's there. This doesn't mean that there is no negativity there, but that our experience is bent over toward the pleasant. We can go around then talking about loving feelings, about how good we feel about everything and everyone: maybe we have a tee-shirt with the words over the chest, Love everyone. We can go around that way if we want.

But the first thing is to experience; then the talk will follow the experience.

45

We can see a preference, thinking that the way out of something unpleasant is by steering out of it. When we clearly see the process of avoidance, attentiveness is present; the not looking at a "problem" is looked at. Looking has moved in where there was avoidance of looking! Going around our present situation becomes a going through it! Then we can go through to the other side; not getting stuck in the unpleasantness, but not avoiding it, either.

This is going on beyond conditioning, not by avoiding conditioning, but by going through conditioning.

We let what is happening in our present life show itself to us. So this going through conditioning has a very simple aspect: it takes no plan. No plan of ego is required, no plan of ego is appropriate to end ego. Ego is not going to do that. While ego is operating, its own effort, its own tendency, is towards strengthening its own pattern, however it accomplishes that. Perhaps it uses fear: Yes, here's a danger. I'd better stay out of this situation. I can't take this at all! If we listen to such a train of thoughts, we strengthen our conditioning. That's the way fear works.

Going beyond conditioning does not take fighting conditioning. We simply see here that conditioning isn't the whole picture, the whole reality. We see that conditioning will tend to maintain itself, to keep things as comfortable as possible, stable, within its own limits.

While we are watching conditioning, we have an opportunity to look into ourselves, into our pains. We do not merely see that something involves pain for us: Indeed, if we see only that there is pain, we do not see the full reality. We can also see the specific things that are bothersome to us, how they work, how they bother us, how we are bothered.

When we start out as the fish, all that we see are the specifics of our conditioned existence. In the process of watching these specifics of our conditioned existence, we naturally come to see the limits, the edges, the borders, the boundaries of this conditioned existence. Through the experience of the conditioned comes the appreciation of the non-conditioned. This appreciation is the space in which the conditioned can be, in which it can be easily allowed to be. This space is like an island which is unbothered by waves beating against the shore, like a cool spot under a shade tree which is not overheated by a broiling sun. It is a way of experience that *allows* conditioning, without putting energy into that conditioning. So the conditioning has only *its* old momentum, but no new energy. With patience we can see its momentum diminish, like a once-roaring fire that has not been fed new branches and is now only embers.

This process of letting painful conditioned patterns roll down to a stop, or burn out, involves our patience. And, with our continual attention, there is little energy if any feeding the conditioning processes now on the wane. Still, this is not a picnic.

Or maybe it is. If we can have a picnic, or not have a picnic, we are free to have a picnic when life is a picnic for us, and free not to when it isn't.

VIPASSANA SHMIPASSANA

It may dawn on you that vipassana isn't so great. That it is a waste of time. That there is no value in formal sitting practice, nor in there being a meditation centre. At least, definitely not in a way personally involving you. Then we can hear ourselves ask the question of Why do any more sitting, or Why stay at the meditation centre any longer. This may lead to conclusions—thoughts or images about starting some other activity: standing up, or travelling away from the centre. We may see ourselves decide to drop out of the vipassana scene altogether. What was this vipassana supposed to do, anyway? Did it once actually have some appeal?

Do we feel ashamed to ask such questions, or defiant? Such questions may strike us as heretical. Or as disrespectful. Or, put a Buddhist way, as a manifestation of "Ignorance". So we may put these questions aside as worthless or bad in some sense. We see that feelings can be suppressed this way. Done in the lofty name of Buddhism, perhaps, but still a way of suppression.

Can't we just transcend Buddhist concepts for a minute, and accept how we feel?

Let's allow questioning. Questioning irritates the dogmatic mind and frustrates the desire for certainty. Questioning clears out mental drowsiness. It energises our alertness. It leads to deep insight. The greater the doubt, as some put it, the greater the satori.

In the questioning mind is the natural tendency to investigate our present situation. This is the way of discovery through the presence of mindfulness on a practical level.

When we see this questioning, what is it, really, that is being questioned? There is some image or concept of a practice here, and a dissatisfaction with that practice: it isn't producing what we wanted! Hey! I've been doing vipassana for almost a decade now, and I still (fill in your own rut here)!

Disappointed expectations. Impatience. Troublesome times. Something in our trip through human existence we aren't content about.

Are we fighting our situation? Well, what *is* our situation? Do we identify our dissatisfaction as "vipassana"!? Come on now, really!! Are we angry at an idea (!) for our continuing life, an all-too-human existence? Imagine that! Did we really think, imagine, that life would stop going through its changes, its challenges, just because we sit still a few hours a day, or live in a community of "spiritually" oriented friends, perhaps among "high" and "developed" individuals? This imagination of ours is supplying us here with distractions and scapegoats to defuse later frustrations, isn't it?

In any case, here we still are. Even the Buddha grew old and died. Life hasn't stopped going through its changes here either. Will our imagination lead us to focus our dissatisfaction here on a sitting practice, or on the quality of a community, or on those individuals who *must* be, after all, not really so high and developed?

This sees the animation of our own life processes as coming from outside, over there somewhere. When we are this way and we notice joy, happiness, loving feelings, we may feel gratitude for the Teaching. Or, for the teacher. And when we notice misery, dejection, hate, we may feel resentful against the limits of this, after all, not so wonderful Teaching. Or, of the teacher! This is like breaking a mirror for what we see in it.

It doesn't matter if we follow this mirror-breaking way of dealing with our situation or not. It doesn't matter if we stop the practice of sitting meditation; if we leave a meditation centre. (This is *not* to say that it makes no difference.) In either case, we have ourselves with us. In either case, life goes on. In either case, life's concerns are still there for us to deal with.

Check it out for yourself. Isn't it so? And *if* so, where do *you* go from here!

DO WHAT TEACHES

Do what teaches.
Leave behind what reteaches what you already know.
Watch energy born of fear, worried energy, energy for keeping us
    in place, for locking out the unknown.
Dive into the void.

Learning to face what is difficult, we come to see what brings along
something strikingly unpleasant, painful, with it.

We see what the whole situation calls for, rather than focusing on
    what we happen to want at the moment.

We travel through all sort of spaces, experiences, situations, using
    whatever comes along to grow from, to learn through, to
    appreciate. Thenit doesn't matter much what it is specifi-
    cally which comes along. We become a chameleon that lets
    itself be fully absorbed into each experience, in sympathy
    with each new situation, and yet the chameleon goes on.
    There is this resonating, this sympathizing, in experience
    more and more deeply.

RECOLLECTIONS

Recollections of
    the you you were and the way they saw you as,
    the beliefs you held,
    the feelings you felt.
Just recollections.
You don't know yourself anymore—
Live and learn.
        Open-eyed, just seeing what is,
        grounded in awareness,
        grounded anywhere,
        grounded everywhere.
Groundless traveler always at home.

WHERE'S THE LOVE IN VIPASSANA?

Q. Vipassana Meditation seems one-sided to me, lacking in love. How does love, the heart, come into Vipassana practice? *I can't see it!*

A. Yes, how does the heart come into Vipassana? You may feel Vipassana is dry and cold. Or that may be your experience now in meditation: that there are no feelings of love in the present moment. And under all of that, there is a valuing of the Way of the Heart. We can look and see if we have an image of Vipassana here, a desire or a demand for it to be something specific, or to do something specific for us.

We can understand that Vipassana Meditation is not a particular feeling or emotion or psychological state or physical state. It is no particular experience at all. It has no given form. It is just a space in which we have the possibility of seeing whatever it is that comes to us in life.

This space Vipassana may allow us to see love, if we are feeling love. It may allow us to see the limit to love, if the love we are aware of has a limit. The space itself is neither the fullness, nor the limit, of love. We can appreciate that.

What is central here is the valuing of the Way of the Heart, the Way of Caring, which underlies this uneasiness about Vipassana practice. Yet we can see that this empty space of mindfulness is bringing you more deeply in touch with your own compassionate nature.

Can you see it now?

GROWTH THROUGH LOVE

Love can make us grow. Do we have this type of love between us and those we love? Do we relate in a way that allows for expansion and growth in depth—for the other we feel we love, and for ourselves?

We sometimes relate in a critical, unaccepting way. We want something from the other person which is not forthcoming. This can lead to a feeling of hurt or rejection which can in turn lead to a defensive withdrawal or to a defensive attacking. Then the other often responds by not accepting *our* unaccepting stance.

But we can each go on now to simply seeing what the other is experiencing and how the other is changing. We have no need to withdraw or to attack when we see fully and acknowledge *deeply*, first of all to ourselves, and then to the other, what we see. This is *called* being accepting. It is simply the perception of what is happening, and allowing it to resonate for us, in us.

Then we can gently guide ourselves, and one another, to a more accepting, expansive, courageous, more welcoming frame of mind.

SPIRITUAL RELATIONSHIP

What makes a relationship spiritual, we might guess, is that in it we are relating to something spiritual, something divine, godly, or other-worldly. I want to suggest, rather, that in it we are relating to something spiritually. It is a matter of *how* we relate, rather than of *what* we relate to. It is a matter of attitude.

This attitude allows us to relate as an ally in the exploration of life. How do we become allies with those we relate to? By coming to the other with the awareness that we are fellow travellers, fellow experiencers of the onflowing show, and by treating ourselves and the other as centres of life: with caring and open curiosity and wonderment. An ally is there sharing and exchanging feelings, observations, reactions, experiences in general. This caring curiosity, which leads to sharing, leaves behind the demanding curiosity of an opponent looking for ways to attack and criticise. The ally lives out the "spiritual" attitude; this attitude is a loving one, one which leads to confident trust and openness.

This attitude makes for an evolution, a growth, an expansion—one which is possible in the context of a relationship with another person; in fact, not only *in* this context but growing out of this context itself. This context is love.

Love is deep heart-felt friendship-in-action. Love is not a passively felt sensation, like a twitching or an ache, but an attitude. And it is an attitude in practice: it is an attitude which is carried into action, an attitude with ongoing manifestations. It is not merely an attitude simply held as a doctrine or a credo.

Love is having the beloved's well-being at heart. When this is based on an appreciation of what is happening for the beloved, and is free from conflicting needs or demands of our own egos, this love can operate beneficiently for the beloved.

Love is flexibility, allowing ourselves to be open to and responsive to the needs and yearnings of the beloved. Love is not stubborn, not rigid, not prideful. It is miraculous: The more we give love, the more love we have. For in giving love, as in making (creating) love, we experience love, and the more we experience love, the better we know it, and the more its vitality glows through all our body. Loving the beloved, giving our love to the beloved, acting for the beloved, rejuvenates the lover as much as it satisfies the beloved. It enrichens both. It is what makes us rich human beings. And its absence? Well, what *is* a person who feels no love in the heart? A poor, sombre, joyless presence, wouldn't you say?

53

SHIVA FRIENDSHIP

I shall play the wind, to your butterfly. Let me lift you to the sky; your flips and turns and rolls and drops let me guide. Invisible to all the others, you will feel my presence, embracing your every move through space.

I shall play the star, to your star. Let me twinkle back to you as we shine on. Light years apart, we will be visible to one another, even when clouds darken the skies to all the others.

I shall play the non-intruder, to your lover. Let me feel your developing love for one another, know the growing intensity between you two, remain apart while you go where you know not.

I shall play the ineffable, to your silence. Beyond all words, beyond om, beyond, I shall abide in quiet. Waves let us accept, moving through us, neither ignored nor disturbing.

TROUBLES IN RELATIONSHIP

At times we are alone. Then we see how we feel in aloneness. If we live fully in aloneness, even if we have experiences of loneliness, we are not needy. When we live through aloneness, and deeply appreciate how this affects us, we enter into relationship without a compulsive neediness. Then we can let relationship be.

Relationship involves relating with others, being related to others, being in relation to them, letting them come into us, into our world, and allowing ourselves to enter theirs.

We may find that we enter into relation with another through some idea of relationship. For example, some people seem to be in love with being in love. I want to love someone, they say. Then relating which does occur is under the pressure of how they conceive of a loving form of relationship.

We may have ideas about what relating amounts to.

Or we may have a special idea about what a particular relationship is. This can confine our awareness of the other to the small world which that concept of relationship allows: a man calls his life mate and the mother of his children, Mama. This may have an influence on much of his awareness of this other human being. When there is this influence, this is experiencing through the focused vision of concepts: a mother is just a mother. A mother is not, for example, a person saddened because of some disturbing news. Here our understanding of relationship may blind us: we are bored even when something important is happening, if we are not well aware of it.

Sometimes this relating through our idea can be exciting: this is my lover. This is my long-lost brother. This is my dying granddad. This is my newborn daughter.

This excitement is one more form of Maya. It keeps us, or can keep us, in the world of image, of social fictions, overlooking the reality which is not captured by our thinking. Trying to experience reality through our thinking is like trying to scratch the bottom of our foot through the shoe.

So even when we give ourselves excitement by thinking of what is happening in our relating with another in some specific way, we can be aware that we may be led by this way of thinking to become out of touch with something important. And when we are aware of this tendency, then how we think of our relationship does not delimit what we can be aware of.

When we are simply open to what there is going on, without these ideas closing in our experience, there is a fullness to the moment which is extremely rich, gently poignant, deeply alive. Is it really odd or paradoxical that relating this way, fully, with another human being, without defining that person as having this or that relation to us, can be so deep—even deeper than relating through a concept as seemingly vitalizing as My Darling Lover?

Our thinking about relationship may lead us to set up certain ideals, with which we compare every person we come into contact with. Our idea of a Good Relationship may make extra difficulties for us when we come into conflict, either subtle or gross, with someone we are relating to.

We have never had a fight in the fifty-five years we've been married, she said with contentment and pride. Is this good news? Bad news? Perhaps conflicts between the two were regularly suppressed. Perhaps not.

When conflicts arise in relationship, how are they dealt with? Or do we think that relationships should be without conflict? that they will be, perhaps if the people involved are "harmoniously matched" at least, all milk and honey? Aside from the fact that a diet of only milk and honey might bring on nausea and diarrhoea, *if* it could be had, this ideal defined by lack of turbulence may lead to ill-feelings, to ill-will, if and when turbulences do arrive.

So conflicts may be denied, or avoided: if that's the way you feel, I'll just spend the night playing cards with the boys.

This may "work" for the short term, in that tension may be somewhat lessened when the next day rolls around. We have to see if this is how we want to go through life, never *relating* about the conflicts in relationship. Are these conflicts, part of the very juice of relationship, being treated as an annoying interference with the "real" stuff of it all?

In relationships these conflicts give us the opportunity to appreciate what is difficult for us, and for others. This way leads to greater contact rather than to a cutting off from the other or others involved. We can see our humanity this way. (We are all human beings.) (Or isn't that O.K.?)

56

We notice that with different people these conflicts are dealt with, are responded to, in different ways. Great reactivity may come up in some. Or there may be but little awareness of how each understands what is happening. Of how, according to this understanding, each is feeling about, is evaluating what is happening. Of what each sees as where or how to go on from the present turbulence—*if* anywhere or anyhow.

Sometimes we can appreciate that we are working through some pattern of reactivity. Or seeing into some personality compulsiveness which has been driving us. Or transcending some fear or closedoffness. Or seeing that great, hostile reactivity is the present response to some conflict.

If we are getting slapped around each time a conflict arises, we are dealing with an interpersonal, social (inter-psychological) reality through physical harshness. We can see that some people are handling their frustrations this way. Do we feel that being fully aware of this when it occurs will lead us to end this relation? Or will lead us in compassion to going more deeply into the frustrations these attacks involve? This isn't a matter of one way being the right way and some other way being wrong.

The real value in relationships, in the particular, different forms of relationship which each of us is involved in at any given time, may have nothing to do with our ideas defining what relationships are about. Our ideas don't know. Reality does.

If there is a lot of pain and torment in this relationship, we see how it feels. If we see our energies going into continuing such a painful system, we see how this occurs, what moves our energies in this direction. If our energies are not, we see how this system is either continuing from other energies, or ending on its own.

In this way we see into our own contribution to relationships we are in and how they operate. We see into what we ourselves are like. We see what we like and engage ourselves in.

We may be afraid of noticing some undesirable traits here: I'm mean, or inconsiderate, or selfish, or masochistic. This is identifying with processes which do not feel enriching to us. Such identifying will not hasten these processes to end. If we simply see how things are working, we will know. When we know ourselves we do not know any one, essential *thing*. We simply appreciate how *various* modes of humanity occur, and whether *they* are constricting and poisonous, or expansive and nourishing.

LIBERATING RELATIONSHIP, SPIRITUAL LOVE, PARASAMGATÉ

Have you been involved in relationship these days, or recently? Maybe you've noticed you already have a well-defined idea of what a good relationship is—whether that's a healthy one, or one that's alive, or stimulating, satisfying, expanding, or is it a peaceful one, or one that's fun, therapeutic, or an exciting one? And maybe you've noticed you also already have an idea of a bad one—whether that's a sick relationship, or a neurotic one, or one that's deadening and stagnating, or a peaceful and soporific one, or a fun-and-games superficial one, or a therapeutic and overworked one, or an exciting and agitating, upsetting one.

Whatever ideas we may have, we can look beyond our ideas in order to see what is actually happening for us in our relationships with others.

To start with we may notice that sometimes we feel a pull to a certain relationship, to a certain other person. They catch our attention and appeal to us. And whether we take the relationship to be good or bad, healthy or neurotic, reasonable or incomprehensible, workable or impossible, these certain relations just seem to light up our lives: they just click for us; sometimes *in spite of* ourselves and what we think we want or are looking for: Don't you have this experience ever?

If we notice this, we can see in operation the fact that relationships, as it were, choose us. At least the undeniably powerful ones. They are the ones we can't resist: what they hold for us is too deeply significant for us to deny them or to let them go by.

This means that they are alive for us, that there are certain issues in us which they are relevant to. As some people say, they push our buttons, they give us a buzz, they talk our language, they turn us on.

In this sort of relationship which arises naturally and effortlessly, in a way which feels spontaneous, we can learn a lot about ourselves; not about our *images* of ourselves, but about ourselves.

In relationship we can see how we act, and what our efforts are concentrated on bringing us.

What we are bringing on ourselves in our overall way of being and acting in a relation may of course be strikingly different from what we earnestly think we want in a relationship. This in a way is an astonishing fact. And the source of a lot of pain. Isn't that so? I'm not saying this to lay down a criticism, or to suggest how we *ought* to be in relationship (whatever that way might be), but simply to acknowledge this complication explicitly.

And if there is a source of pain, there is pain. We may not look at what we are driving towards in relation and we may then experience pain. If in this case we direct ourselves into an attack on ourselves or the other as masochistic, we may overlook just how this pain came about. The first thing is to appreciate what's happening. Name-calling doesn't help us to do this.

What we are actually truly involved in in our relationships may not be obvious to us at first, neither what we are working towards there nor what our deepest frustrations are there. In fact, it may take years and decades and many, many similar relationships for us to see these processes clearly.

And we are not working on only one level. So there are a number of these processes, whether satisfying or frustrating to us, to learn about. These are all extremely important lessons for us to learn about ourselves.

What I mean about the difference between what we think we want and are doing in relationship on one hand, and what we are actually moving towards, on the other, may be made clearer by an example.

Terry and Pat meet each other. There is an attraction. They begin to spend time together, and so a relationship is born.

After a while, the two begin to consider the possibility of living together. Anyway, they begin experiencing one another as possible living partners. They feel that their relationship is in the air, on the balance, waiting for their decision. This is how they experience their time together.

Terry thinks that this time together is to allow the two to feel out what being with the other is like, and to allow each to see the other in a more natural, less put-on, less role-playing way. This is for Terry the whole point of the relation here.

And Pat thinks that this time together is to enjoy things together, and go out together, and live in a social world where the two are related to by *other* people as a couple. This is for Pat the whole point of the relation here.

Now an interesting way I have come across to look at the on-going reality of relationships is to ask this question: given how each is vis-à-vis the other, if this relation had been designed to teach each of the two some definite life lesson, what would this lesson be for each of the two?

Now first of all, an outsider may be able to answer this question with no hesitation or doubt, while for the two involved, this may be totally mysterious.

In our example of Terry and Pat, for instance, it may be painfully obvious to friends and others but not to either Terry or Pat, that the great flow of Terry's energy is going towards trying to get Pat to express love and acceptance and tenderness. This is the first observation. And that the great flow of Pat's energy is towards trying to maintain a feeling of control and safety and autonomy. This is also a first observation.

And, to continue, others can make the second observations that Terry is afraid of being deserted or rejected by Pat. And that Pat is afraid of being overpowered or swallowed alive by Terry. And that these two fears provide the energy for how each is acting within the couple.

When the relationship is looked at from this perspective, we see Terry reacting to Pat's distancing manoeuvres, Pat's way of maintaining autonomy: Terry feels slightly rejected and so makes a stronger effort at gaining Pat's love and tenderness. And Pat, feeling more anxious and under pressure, tries harder to keep a neat, separate world where Terry cannot enter. This is a knot which tightens itself on being pulled.

As a tightened knot, the relation is structured to teach *WHAT*?

Each has a chance here, especially if we imagine the attraction and the energy involved here to be great, to see an important aspect of themselves and of one another. There is a golden opportunity for the two to learn about an important fear each has, and how it frustrates the desire of each for contact.

I take it that this is an extremely valuable lesson about themselves, and about one another, for the two to learn.

(This lesson will *not* be learned if the two feel that the only issue is, after all, simply whether to live together or not, and conclude, "No, it's better not to", and let the whole thing drop then and there!)

Terry may come to see in looking further, for example, what acting on the fear of rejection brings about where the other person responds by becoming more distant or colder. And Pat may come to see what trying to keep well separated from another brings about where the other person responds by driving for more closeness.

These are important *first* lessons. Each may well learn the way their typical or "characteristic" or so-called natural—referring to what is conditioned—way of reacting frustrates them.

And if they (or we) continue to look to see what there is to learn from the relationship, each may come to learn about these fears which constrict and frustrate.

When these fears are stimulated or triggered off by something in the relationship, we (or they) are in a prime position to look into these fears. Often, however, the fear is so strong that we do not find the breathing space to look at it until later. Whenever we can see it is when we can look into what it is about.

FEELING FEAR: there is a movement away from, as an arrow flying into the distance. In going along with fear, we follow the fleeing arrow. If we notice this flight, we may criticize this with an "Oh! We shouldn't have fear!"

This is getting into moralizing. Now, psychologically on the other hand, this fear is a clear indication of something important to us. We can feel that there is something valuable which is being threatened. So what is important to us here? (Flying with the fear can make it more difficult for us to get in touch with what we feel is important here.)

Fear keeps us running. It puts us in a very tight and anxious state of being. When we give ourselves the time and enough room to breathe a little, we can come to know this fear and the related important concern this fear is threatening.

So we can come to see that this fear is based on some strong desire or preference of ours. Terry's fear of being rejected, for example, depends on the desire not to be alone. And Pat's fear of being swallowed depends on the desire to keep constant and still what feels very shaky, wobbly, insecure. Now this looking at *the root desires which underlie fear* leads up in this way to appreciating our own life *experiences* which have deeply marked us. This appreciation can lead to compassion for and understanding of ourselves.

61

And this can give the confidence to look further. (Without confidence, fear is hard to transcend. Hard, not impossible.) Looking further, we come to see what the fear's root, this strong desire, is *itself* resting on. The desire not to be alone, for example, rests on Terry's uncomfortableness at being alone. (This relates, in our example, to powerful experiences in Terry's *past* of anxious and painful aloneness, which condition and perpetuate this *present* fear.) This uncomfortableness may be gone into and through and beyond in pure contemplation, but *it may take the lived reality of being alone for Terry to come face to face with what is uncomfortable* about that for him. (There is also an EERIE attraction to what we fear because we all know just this painful truth!)

One way or another, fear can be seen through. We can see, with investigation or consideration, its intimate relation to our desires and to our wanting to protect ourselves! Imagine learning what self-image is driving us and keeping us the slave of this fear! The key here is an open curiosity about what this self-image really involves us in: how in our *experience* we feel how it structures what we will do or think, and what we will not do or think, how we will feel, and how we will not feel, when we will be at ease, and when we will become anxious. We can experience here how this self-image, a little mental creation we recall from time to time, gives us work and worries, in exchange for a cramped island of apparent safety. (Watch out it doesn't sink, or get invaded, or even lost.) Then we are seeing in reality how we truly feel when deeply identifying with or clinging to or being saddled with a given fear-generating self-image. When we do *that* enough, it will be time to just let it all drop!!!

Until we get to these roots of the fear in our desires and self-concerns and images, we do not fully see or experience or understand this fear. When we do see these roots and work through what they (don't be misled) do for us, when we are no longer boxed into what they "help" us avoid, then we have been thorough in our uprooting and we *have* worked through what they are about, and *are* through. Being thorough, we go and are through, thoroughly through: in a Sanskrit chant this process was celebrated with "gaté (going), gaté (going), pāragaté (going through, past, and beyond), pārasamgaté (going completely beyond)".

And when we are through in this way, this fear is no longer able to take root in us. Then the fear cannot drive us blindly along anymore as it had been doing up until then.

At that stage in our learning about and "working through" our conditioning, we can see the fear arise, see what triggers it off, and simply let it be, not having it lead us even one little bit, totally inconsequential, neither binding nor frustrating.

This is freedom from specific fears through working through their roots in our self-imposed strictures created by our karma, our past actions and reactions to life's situations. When these strictures/structures are seen and let be to burn out ("burning karma": karma which is burning out), we have seen ourselves and our fears and their end. And it is each specific relationship which can show us ourselves and our fears. (And can show us all the rest, too, of course.)

We can say here that each such relationship then gives us the key to freeing ourselves a little. This is when relationship frees us from our self-defeating patterns: liberating relationship.

The self-discovery which underlies this becoming free is most powerful when there is a strong and undeniable attraction between the two in spite of these self-defeating, or rather, frustrating, patterns. This attraction becomes a spotlight which makes it possible to see the frustrating patterns in greater highlight than usual. This may be used to see these more deeply, and to go more fundamentally beyond these patterns. This strong attraction is a liberating force. Do you remember when we were troubadours, and would pass the word about this liberating force by singing of Spiritual Love?

I LOVE YOU

I love you where there is no language : in the silence where we two see all realities in their flow. We look together and see what is going by and accept all there is to accept, which is, all there is, all. If we touch by means of the body-sense, it is not *in order to* BECOME close : we are already one : we have already been through some of the same spaces of consciousness. We have looked at each other, and seen—beyond all manifestation, beyond each moment of consciousness—the other, resting open and loving, fully accepting, fully understanding, fully feeling, sensing, and thinking. We look at each reality as it is, not belonging to anyone—even thoughts of This is mine. You bring to me, for me to see, a light of life, and there is joy in the seeing of this visible energy. The light is ownerless. It goes through "our" awareness : you are illuminating, my shining being, my deva, and you are neither within or without. In joy and love I lower my head towards you, and I say Namas te.

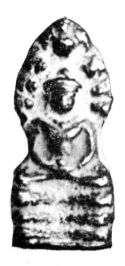

Nāga-Buddha-rūpa
XI-XIVth Century
Lopburī Style
Thailand

To The Beloved, Ishq'allah, Krishna, Holy YOU

I live in YOU breathe me
              in
              and out
              and in I live through YOU nourish me
                            YOUR energy
gives me life I grow in joy
              feeling YOU in me, YOU
                      before me, YOU
                      around me, YOU
YOU
        are limitless
           energy itself
           life in form
              in flow
                  changing
                  growing
                  evolving
                      the beauty of life.
THIS totality-in-movement
        full
                  answering all demands effortlessly
                      with what already manifests
                            YOU.

HEART-FELT THINKING

Breathing is on-going: at times it is shallow, at times deep; at times brief, at times long; sometimes silent, and other times audible. Watching these changes, we are continually aware of our body. If we keep feeling the expansion and contraction in our chest area, where the lungs are filling and emptying, we are more in touch with our body's relation to what is happening at each moment.

It's all in the breathing. Being grounded in movement, non-statically, comes with experiencing the present reality through our bodies. An aspect of this is being in constant touch with how our bodies are. When there is a tightness in the heart area, constricting breathing, something is tension-producing in the moment. We can experience such a tension without rejecting our experience, without trying to make our bodies relax, without *wanting* our bodies to be relaxed, simply noticing the tension, accepting it fully, welcoming it as highlighting for us some dissatisfaction.

Or perhaps the breathing is slow and deep. Do we see the ease in the moment? Then we can be fully alive to the harmonious situation.

At times we are experiencing life from within our heart area. At other times, we are trying to figure out what is happening. The latter gives us headaches, especially above or in the eyes, while the former centres us with heart-felt awareness. So, staying with our heart area, we are not channelling our life's energies here into cerebral processes; we are simply feeling with our full being what is happening. This is not constricting the depths of our "being in touch with reality" to what we can comprehend, can understand, but giving full reign to *all* of our prowess as sentient beings.

Then there is a clearly experienced harmony between our thinking and our full feeling. We can call this thinking with the heart, heart-felt thinking.

>   As you breathe in
>   As you breathe out
>   When there is no breathing—
>   what's happening in your heart?

*

67

ANGER AND ILL-WILL

Sometimes we would rather believe anything than acknowledge certain realities, than experience certain emotions. We want life to be pleasant. We retract from tensions and from what we fear will be painful. We complicate our lives at times in this attempt at peacefulness.

We want not to be upset. We want things not to bother us. We want not to get riled up. This leads to a frustration when we start to become upset, when things do begin to bother us.

We don't want to cause waves. We don't want to confront others. We'd like to be a nice chap or a nice lady. We swallow our irritation, our annoyance, our resentment. We try to feel pure and above anger. Afraid to face our emotions, afraid to express our displeasures, afraid to stand up for ourselves, we hide behind the distorting self-image of an evolved or spiritual or holy being. We talk of the sin or of the 'unskilful' nature of ill-will, of anger. Inside we seethe with rage, or stew in irritation. Outside we are very pleasant, indeed. This is not evolved or spiritual or holy. It is simply putting on a façade which makes it more devious for us to come to see ourselves as we truly are.

We might feel that anger is agitating and unpleasant, and believe that it ought to be suppressed, or that we should be above it. Or we might feel that anger is healthy, and believe that it ought to be expressed, or that we should get into our anger and encourage it along.

What I have noticed is that on some occasions anger is expressed, even explosively, and that nonetheless it is not cleaned out by this process. And on other occasions, anger is not expressed but dealt with in a complete way even so. I feel that the essential issue is not whether we get into being demonstrative in our anger or not, but whether we recognize the anger, acknowledge it readily, and experience it, its roots, its manifestations, all fully and consciously, or not.

In anger we can experience a visceral and emotional response to something which infringes on our freedom of action or on our sense of well-being. Anger itself, we can see, is the manifestation of a stand in the world. This may be lauded or criticized or may simply be seen for what it actually is.

In ill-will we can experience a mental attitude. Perhaps we can see the frustration or sadness underlying this critical mentality, which may itself be focused or may be diffusely applied against whatever comes to our attention. It frequently feels rancorous or festering within us. We may come to appreciate that not acknowledging and consciously experiencing anger may result in a build-up of ill-will and resentment. In Pali, this state is described by the word paṭigha (Skt. pratigha) meaning literally striking (-gha) back against (paṭi-, prati-). Some of you may perhaps be reminded here of Nietzsche's incisive words on ressentiment, this all-too-common phenomenon of impotent rage (*Geneology of Morals*, Part I).

If there is anger, we have the possibility of feeling the energy of this state, the feeling of groundedness or of agitation which accompanies it, our confidence or our cowardice.

If there is ill-will, we can see what it is which we find unacceptable, what we want to be different, what we resent. Here we have the opportunity to see how ill-will arises, how it affects our thoughts, our responses to others, our bodies. We can see the critical orientation it gives to our perception, and the bitter flavour it gives to our experience.

When we get inside anger, or inside ill-will, not to identify with them 'Oh, that's what I'm like', but simply to experience the phenomena occurring to us, we can learn more about ourselves, about our desires and their frustrations, and about how we deal with that unhappy reality. And we can see when they go, how they go, whether we chase them away, suppress them, or whether we allow them to show themselves fully to us, be heard, and leave of their own accord when finished.

LIVING THROUGH FEAR

It's all changing. That's nothing new. But even *how* it's all changing feels different—the magnitude of changes is increasing, isn't it, all over the world. Impermanence, or anicca, even in anicca. Now we can experience not only velocity, change through time, but also acceleration, changes in change through time! And where's it all going?

Things seem to many to be beyond control, to be heading rapidly in a disastrous direction. Species seem to be dying off almost daily. Anyone who reads a newspaper or tunes in to a news programme even occasionally is almost painfully aware of such trends.

In times like this, there will be much fear to experience. Fear leads to freezing up, to searching for safety, to fantasies of better days gone by: nostalgia, perhaps to high circus by way of manicked avoidance of the "heavies", of the great pain all around, lurking almost everywhere. There is much more to fear than fear itself, as any sampling of people in fear will show.

Fear rests on confusion, and on ego concerns. Its drive is towards unseeing action, wherever that might lead from the particular situation in which it arises. Its overcoming is through patience: the patience to remain where the fear is, to accept the confusion, the unseeing, and to keep on the path, to keep on watching at every moment to see better into this not-yet-clear, problem-filled reality.

This isn't a nice matter of "perfecting one's paramis or paramitas" as part of any idealized diversion, but of coming full-face to grips with what we wish were different.

We can see into fear by looking at what is *easy* to observe— perhaps this is day-dreaming's wishes and imaginings. Through these we can experience how we conceive or imagine a "better" reality to be. If we allow the imagination full reign, and look into what *most* appeals to us, we can continue to see, through *this* extreme, what *least* appeals to us in this present situation, experienced as either itself horrible or implying some horrible future.

In any case, there is no choice here. The present is what it is. Greatly difficult times are times of great opportunity for gaining in understanding, in patience, in love, in magnanimity.

In Buddhist terms, it is through suffering through *all* of Mankind's woes that the way out of each and every one of them is

70

seen, and thereby can a bodhisattva be of deepest aid to all other sufferers. The bodhisattva vow to save an infinite number of beings from suffering is a wonderful but so deep, so immense a commitment when what it truly involves is appreciated. Homage to all Buddhas, to all Arahats, homage to all Bodhisattvas, and homage to all of us.

FROM FEAR TO OPEN FRIENDSHIP

We all want love and the good companionship of others, at least occasionally. Or, at least many people will readily admit to such desires.

Is there anyone who would not like warm, loving feelings, caring about one another, being alive to the joys and sorrows of friends, being filled with love, admiration, concern, good-will?

Yet, even so, this isn't the way it always turns out. In spite of our desires.

So why is this so? We may have the good fortune to be able to share the open company of others. Can we look, though, when it happens, to see what gets in the way of this easy sharing?

Are we alert enough to hear what the other is saying, not so much in the words, but deep down? Do we realize how the other is feeling, what frame of mind he or she has at the moment?

Perhaps we do. Yet we *still* might find, much to our dismay or at least to our surprise, that we seem to turn quickly away from this appreciation of the other to a less intimate, less in-touch awareness, and so, to a less intimate, less in-touch communication.

We may begin debating with what was said. Or we may simply express *our* understanding or appreciation of what is being talked about.

Or we may go from that appreciation to some old situation which that brings to mind.

Are we aware that our body has pulled back from our companion? That it is getting more tensed?

Have we returned to our own reality? Was this simply keeping centred, or non-distracted? Or perhaps we notice an element of distance from the other person, of wanting to make sure that it's clear to everyone, especially to ourselves, how *we* think, how *we* feel—in short, who *we* are.

So this concern to stay in touch with ourselves may limit our openness to others.

The way out of this is not through developing self-hatred because we are closed off to others.

What there is to see is this: a feeling of insecurity, of being unsure of ourselves, of wanting to be assured of who we are. Do we look below these uneasy feelings, to see what they rest on?

Can we see fear at all? Fear about who we are? (There can be such fear even if there is no "me", no "you".) We may *experience* this as a fear, worry, minor concern, occasional issue, that others won't like us, like who we are, like what they "know" of us, like what they see of us.

This can show itself at other times when we notice ourselves *worrying* about what to wear, or how we look ("Do I look O.K., honey?"), or in other ways.

We can look into this type of fear and so meet up with our ideas about what we *should* be like, and trembling nervously behind this, our ignorance or false "knowledge" about who we are. Once we can see the self-image that we are taking to be a reality worrisome and unacceptable, once we can see who it is we fear we really are, we can begin looking through this image—first to see how it is influencing, perhaps even controlling, our thoughts, our actions, much of our life's energies; and then, to see *its* roots

Uprooting cannot occur unless force is applied at the base of the tree. And so, this crippling pattern cannot be uprooted unless we are at *its* base. But as it does get uprooted, we go naturally from fear to open friendship.

Can you taste the sweet fruits of this investigation? Can you feel, right now, the worth of this digging? Acknowledging this feeling deeply will give energy to the investigation; the only tool required is timely attentiveness to ourselves in each of the situations life provides for us.

WE'RE ANGRY

We're angry at others now for what we fear we might be like.

We see all of the torment, the dukkha, our worries about who we really are lead to. Attempts at self-definition too are passing mental processes, arising out of this or that. No reason to clutch on to these processes, these attempts. We let go; we let them go by. No self; no worry about self-image.

Self-image : mirage of a delusion.

No self-image; no fears, worries, anxieties about who we are.

Time to end self-doubt is when issue of self and self-definition or essential nature arises, whenever it arises, then and there.

We can be feeling how people are rather than merely understanding what they (their words) are saying.
The mind's limit is the imagination; the heart's, fear.
If I misunderstand you, I end up confusing myself.
The mind's knowing is knowledge; the heart's, understanding.
In deep relationship comes fullness of heart not fullness of self.

THE PASSIONATE BUDDHIST

There are *levels* of "open mindfulness": Have we allowed ourselves to feel our own depths, the degree to which we are capable of resonating in harmony with our environment? Do we appreciate our own richness?

When we let go of our controlling, and let our situation and ourselves in that situation, become fully intermeshed, we are in for the experiences of our lives! All of this is extremely powerful: to be completely alive is the farthest thing from boredom there is.

As we let go, either bit by bit, aspect by aspect, level by level, or radically, all at once—watch what happens.

We stop demanding to know everything in advance. We are no longer sure of where things will go before they go there. We have no solid footing.

But we still have awareness of where things are when they are there (here). We can see our own reactions to our not feeling in control. We know in our heart and in our gut how we feel at the moment.

Here we just appreciate how our changing situation is making us feel, and what we do here in dance, in interaction, with our situation.

We see into our moods. Once controlled and moderated, they may well look like ocean swells where once there were only creek ripples. It's all full of vitality. We do not have to adjust this, to get back to a "middle path". Our fully experiencing each swell ends at the levelling out and ending of each swell. Or did we take on the idea that unless we ended a feeling it would just go on for ever? Then we will be surprised by its ending on its own.

In this continual alertness and full allowing acceptance of our being and reacting, whatever they are like, there is a great stability. This is not the stability of a tin man at attention, but of a ripe, mature, flexible human who can feel (ein echter Mensch: a *real* human).

Once we know what it is to be fully alive, the model of an individual who takes care never to do anything ("Watch out that you don't create any more karma") and who is neutral to everything that happens ("Be without desire") has little appeal. Why choose a puddle-life when life's energies are oceanic?

What a joy to be alive. What wonders are life itself, consciousness and awareness, contact between living beings! How magnificent when we dare to live fully, to be open to all of reality (not merely to what fits our model of some "correct" or even "enlightened" life).

Here we feel creative, light, flexible, alert, energized, clear, open to life's possibilities. We are no longer fasters at the feast.

We thrive on the changes we experience. We see how reality moves on, coming to fruition effortlessly when we do not try to hold it back. Each stage goes deeply through us. We *live* through each, fully, deeply.

Full living is not for the weak-hearted!

DEATH-CANAL LIFE-THROWS

Not enough air. Gasping. Still not enough. One of these exhalations will be followed by no inhalation! Sensation will go slowly, little by little, then blindness, numbness, deafness, death: Wait!!

So long as the task is to keep away the full face of death, when this body will cease inhalations, will take its last sigh, and respire no more—so long will this work have to fail, *some* day.

What is it to be about to die and say, Wait!! I can't die yet! When the child is moving down between your legs and the muscles from the top of your head are flowing down in stepwise contractions toward your toes, what is it to try to stop that! And what, when your bowels want to empty themselves and in their contractions force whatever masses there are within them down toward and through their opening, what is it to try to stop that!

Childbirth and defecating could be lessons—the latter much more available—on how to see that those processes which are occurring are simply occurring. Imagine facing death with that seeing.

As was said, the important thing in life is to learn how to die. Now, since bravery is a bold front in face of something terrifying, this lesson is not: to learn to die bravely; but, rather: to learn not to need to die bravely.

THE HEART PULLS US ON

The heart pulls us on to live.
How can we refuse it?
By being heartless.

Half-hearted, I rest alone. It is only a transient stage. My fulfilment lies in the summer of rebirth, when I become you. 'Til then I am jealous most of all of you, who are always close to you.

How does the heart open?
Sometimes it's so intense, with chest-shaking sobbing, and then, blam! the detonation of an explosive in the heart of the chest. And then—a deep relaxing of all chest muscles, and in the whole body; and a glowing peace. The all-open calm. A golden radiating from the heart of the chest outwards into the arms. Returning to the place of peace filling all of the chest cavity.
Sometimes it is a very easy and nonstrained and gentle process: like the melting of snow on a warm spring day.

The heart pulls us on to live.
How can we refuse it?
By being heartless.

THE STINGY HEART

The heart without a feeling of love, with no joy, is so sad. But, still, we can bear to look at it. Then we can see what it is to feel without love.

Oh, I am so worthless. No one likes me. Or at least, no one with any reasonable values likes me. We can notice that in this state of mind we feel unworthy, and we expect others to feel the same towards us. We look down, or away, unwilling to look at the hatred we think we would see if we looked. So our feeling of isolation increases by our taking this passing thought, feeling, expectation to be reality.

We can notice that we tighten the chest, or pull the head down and in to close the chest, or bring the shoulders forward, or cramp the belly space. All this makes us feel unexpansive and uncomfortable on the physical level. And the feeling on the psychological or emotional level is no different, is it?

I want to hold on to the little love I feel. So we do just that. Stingy with love.

If we have little money and we hoard it, at least it won't diminish.

And if we do give it away, we *will* have less than the little we began with.

When we act this way with our feeling little love, we can see, we can experience, that love is very unlike money.

The more we close our love in, the less love we feel, the less love we *have*.

When *do* we feel love in our hearts? Is it when love is coming in to our empty heart? If we feel a lack of love in our hearts, love coming in to us may only make us feel worse, or, more numb. Oh, *they* are so loving; I am so much colder than they are. That's thinking typical of such a frame of mind, isn't it?

Do we feel love in our hearts when we are possessive about love, when we grab at whatever love comes to us? When we want and feel a need for love, and love comes to us, is it *ever* enough? Do we feel that the *stinginess* of love is in the *other* person, the one being loving towards us?

This may lead us to *demand* love; to feel this desire and this need for more love, and to think that others, or certain particular others, *ought* to give it to us, or, at least to hope and to pray that these others *will* give us this love.

We want others to give us love; we want to hold on tight to the little love we feel; we think that this will bring us peace.

The stingy frame of heart with its demand for a favourable balance of trade in the love market will not reach peace.

So, again let us ask, when *have* we felt love in our hearts? We can look here into our own experiences. How have we felt towards others at such times? We can see that the more love we gave out towards others, the *larger* our own heart felt, the warmer.

Yet, following the mechanical rule, the idea, Give love to others to feel love in your heart, is to give ourselves a task, an obligation. This may well lead to feelings of failure, resentment, anger, rancour, bitterness. We can't mechanically give love. If it flows forth, it flows forth. If it doesn't, we can see that it doesn't. There's an obstacle to the flow here, then.

The place to look for greater love in our hearts isn't especially in how *we* are lovable, especially when we feel unlovable. At such times we can still see what touches our heart for those, in those, we have contact with.

This takes going beyond ourselves. When we feel so miserable, the tendency is often to shut off to everything outside ourselves. So we can gently lift our awareness, with good-willed energy, to the rest of reality at such times.

What will we experience then? Sadness? Anger? Fear? Love? If we look, we will appreciate our relatedness to the rest of reality and how that relating is working, and how it is all resonating in our hearts.

SOFT ARE YOUR WAYS

Soft are your ways
and loving.
Few are your words but full of truth,
spoken from the heart.
Gentle and shy
I feel you reach out,
gingerly,
with love.
You are precious to me
My friend.

PHYSICAL LOVE

Touching.
Holding.
Cuddling.
Breathing
as one.
Flowing motion;
full harmonies.
Bodies
in
musicless
dance,
neither leading,
both alive with
movement.
Rhythms
of the
Universe.
Mystical
Union.

MEMORY IN THE PRESENT

Sometimes old memories are a gentle reminder, if we do not refuse them full entry into our consciousness, of some past still burning at our soul/psyche/mind/being. The advice to Let go, to Stay in the present, is well-intentioned as a *balance* against incessant obsessing. But this Be here now! advice can sway over gently, or not gently, into Cut off thoughts of the past! Then it has become still one more means of repression, of trying to censor certain awarenesses from our consciousness. If we can allow the past's reappearance in, when *it* shows up, we are not clinging to it, but we are also not expending energy in fighting the memory out of consciousness. Then we can see that this energy is otherwise usefully channelled into merely looking.

To let it be gone when it isn't there, but to learn as much as we can see when it does show up, feels like a gentle balance, don't you agree?

Some insistent memories are from times when it felt that things were happening too fast to take in, so that there were experience gaps. Recollection allows us to fill in these gaps so that they can *truly* be done with. In this process we notice an experiencing now of what earlier was too intense or too painful to live fully at the time. So we let ourselves move onwards at the rate we best operate at. There's no inner battle that has to be set up by turning this matter of moving onwards into an ideal about how to change. To accept our own rhythms, to appreciate them, is to see their divine beauty.

Do we fight memory ideas, or future-imagining ideas? I am reminded of some words from ages ago:

> If you wish to move in the One Way
> do not dislike even the world of senses and ideas.
> Indeed, to accept them fully is identical with
> true Enlightenment.

(from a little talk called "Verses on the Faith Mind", *Hsin Hsin Ming*, by the third Zen Patriarch, Seng-ts'an, following the translation of Richard Clarke).

THE PAST

What is the past? Perhaps it is all that has come and gone. All that has been and is now done with. Or perhaps the past is that which lingers on, haunting us. It may be that which keeps us from being newly alive at each moment.

We may feel that certain incidents in our lives will stay with us no matter how old we become. Or that certain patterns of acting are engrained in us until death. That we are nothing but the product of our past, perhaps of only our first few years. Is the past what we are trapped in?

Or perhaps the past is an old friend we return to for comfort and calm companionship. An alternative to the unfamiliar, the strange.

We all know the experience of going back to some event from the past, of recollecting something. And then, either an instant or an hour later, of the jolting experience of snapping abruptly out of that memory.

So something is alive from the past. Something is unsettled.

How do we treat this remembering when it occurs? We may just let it arise and come into awareness. Then it is *merely* noticed. When there is a memory-thought, there is just thinking. Or there may be a feeling of dissatisfaction which arises then, the feeling of having done something wrong. Oh, I've lost it again! I think too much! When we look back at what has been happening and respond this way, we are on a self-evaluating trip, criticising ourselves.

If we can notice that there is some resistance to the natural, spontaneous process of having a memory arise, we can more clearly see what the memory is and what the resistance is. Is there just recollecting? Or does the command come to you, Hey you! Be here now! Have you taken on the rule not to remember anything? Then surely you will break your rule. A wise general never gives a command to the troops which they cannot carry out.

So perhaps we *do* want not to have *any* memories arise. But this is definitely a *specific* memory coming up here, anyway. The memory arises. So there was once an experience. And this is resulting now in something coming up to us in consciousness. We can look at this recollection with our present attentiveness. We see how it *now* affects us, how we have changed since that experience actually occurred. So these recollections from the past will give us material we can clear up from time to time.

When we see a memory arise, can we see it for what it is? We can acknowledge it to be a recollection while knowing that the reality which it conjures up is no more.

If we look carefully when a memory arises, we can see some feeling accompanying that memory. Having the memory arise may be pleasant, or uncomfortable for us, or neutral. This feeling, whatever it is, is the key to the *present* status of the memory. So we must be quite attentive to noticing its flavour and texture. We can greatly increase our understanding if we stay with this accompanying feeling. It is stuffed with information for us about the *present: It may be the recollection of some PAST event but it is a PRESENT recollection.*

When we stay with this accompanying feeling, we appreciate its intensity. Perhaps it begins as a very weak feeling. Perhaps it has an even surface but develops strong undercurrents, say, of joy. We perhaps see an inner satisfaction arise about what we have done. Can we accept this joy, this satisfaction? We *can* notice here the basis of this joy or satisfaction. Do we see what we are joyous or satisfied about, what about ourselves is pleasing or satisfying to us?

Or, as the memory ends, there may arise, for example, a bitter aftertaste. Is it clear then what is disagreeable to us? We can focus in here on what about the memory is unpleasant. We can see what sort of self we now reluctantly experience ourself as. This memory is a remnant from a now-gone past. It may sit heavily on our shoulders and back. Perhaps returning to, being pained by this no-longer-existent "me" is like a habit we can't kick. Are we hooked on a nothing-but-remembered "me"?

Or perhaps we are free of this nothing-but-remembered "me". We are free not in the sense of denying that we did what we did, or that we felt what we felt. But at the same time we can appreciate that *our PRESENT experience is not defined by the past.*

So when a recollection arises, we do not have the attitude, Yes! *That's* me!—There is here neither attraction to the recollection nor aversion to it. We see it arise. We understand its basis, its roots. We know this to be the operation of memory. We know that this recollection can just go by. It is for us a bandwagon we feel no

85

urge to jump on to. It does not make us feel superior to other people because we don't see ourselves in it. It is a ghost town with no one at home. Nor does it make us anxious or at all embarrassed. Why anxiety over some passing thought?

We do not delude ourselves into believing there is something to defend or praise about *anyone* in this process. It is simply a mental process, seen and understood for what it is in its bare nature.

Do you ever have this experience? Can you look for it now sometime? And when we see things clearly this way, the world feels different. The ongoing flow is unobstructed and easy. There is a lack of heaviness. Very agreeable.

So that might be *your* experience of the past we call "yours". But we do not expect all others who have known us, or known of us, to have the same experience. Perhaps you will come across a time when you are free from the past but the person you are with is talking to you as if you *were* that earlier experiencer and doer.

We can see in such a situation whether we are truly free from "our" past. So by meeting up with someone who is responding to our past, we can look to our own experience *just now* to check our own relation to that past. Do we feel annoyance? Perhaps we feel unappreciated in our present form, criticising the other for not noticing us NOW. Are we free from the past in a way which makes us stuck in the present? We may feel an urge to bring the other up to date about us. This *may* simply be easy, open communication. Or it *may* be defensiveness, some form of lack of acceptance. If so, we can look into what about the situation we do not accept; what about the other's stale idea of us we find disagreeable.

People who are feeling that they already know us have a pre-conceived idea of how we act, what we will say, what we will feel. And this idea is at best an accurate overview of our past. Ideas from the past such as these roll onwards with a powerful momentum: This can control present experience if we are not *quite* attentive here. But we can use these ideas and their momentum to learn from. When we are approached by someone who has an idea of us from the past, we can have a liberating meditation. We recall the past they present us with. This does not require us to return to the past patterns at all; nor is letting the past come to us through others a matter of fatalism. We do not have the doctrine: It's my "karma" to live out this scene begun back then. We do not "live it out", for here this living it out would be no different from stay-

86

ing stuck in how we once might have been, or from being pulled back into that pattern. We simply use the other's outdated ideas to help us see more clearly how much we have changed. Mindfulness at such times is essential because of that tendency to return to these earlier painful patterns we call habits or life grooves or life ruts. So perhaps at such times this momentum of theirs *will* drag us back into what we were, leading us into the temptation of acting habitually and blindly.

This outcome, though, is *not* necessary. If we are mindful, we will first perhaps notice a difference between how *we* now feel about things and how the other takes us to be. This should be clearly noted with—and this is crucial—sufficient time spent in this difference to feel its full impact on us. The clearly and fully noting of this is quite powerful. It can stop the shifting back into the old identity of ours which we are being presented with.

Do we just let be the disparity between how *we* now feel and how we are seen? Or do we resist it? In order to stay out of a rut we do not have to do anything, resist anything. All that is appropriate is *lack* of certain action, *lack* of taking the next step in the old rut-sequence.

So we note the disparity. How long do we stay with this? When the situation arises, and you find yourself asking this question, then stay with this disparity a bit longer: See the full reality. What is that reality? We feel that they have not noticed something. That they are not seeing us but just their own earlier-formed image of us. This means we feel there is not true communication going on, and that their ideas are obstructing their perception of the present reality. If so, can we let them have their slowness of perception? Can we let them use their past conceptions in the present? We feel the urge to help them to see with fresh vision.

But we don't have to keep the world up to date about the flow we experience. We can notice, however, whether this idea of bringing the other up to date about us has appeal to us. Do we see *its* roots? Perhaps we feel that if we do not convince the other of how we are different, we will stop being convinced of the change ourselves. Yes, this happens. We may well be afraid of slipping back into an old pain-producing style of ours. We feel that we have recently progressed, but we are shaky and unsure about this progress. This worry or doubt can be looked at. We know now that the way is simply to go on with mindful attentiveness to what is happening. So we can notice, as it begins, this fear of slipping back.

Now we meet up with someone who remembers an old us, and begins relating to us as that old us. We recognise the script. We have gone through this one before, we recall. Do we have stage-fright? Do we feel resistance to going through this again, a fear that we will get stuck in this role being re-assigned to us? Do we want to cut this off? to begin a new play? Perhaps we see a problem to tackle here: to define new conditions for our relating with this person from our past. Do we have an urge to sit down and set up a whole new contract before we go on to anything else? Are we becoming that worried about our slipping back? Let us see clearly. If we are tackling this problem, we are making things quite complicated for ourselves. It's not so hard for us, really: All *we* need is to stay with the ongoing reality. So we recognise this old script. And we see their interest in *starting*, anyway, on that familiar turf. We can accept this interest because we see freshly, in the moment, that it exists. We can unreservedly respond to that interest, with our full, fully-alive awareness. We will be allowing the old script but LIVING FULLY IN ATTENTIVENESS to the *full* interaction occurring between us and the other. For us it will be going into this realm for the first time. As we follow our ever-new awareness, the script subtly changes. We stay on this level. And if the other remains unaware of these subtle changes, our own contact with them is too clear to be blurred for *us*. This requires no fights, no arguments, no debate, no convincing. Surely with mindfulness and patience through time on our parts, the others will ultimately come along on their own, through *their own observations*.

In this way the realisation by others of how we are now different will come about simply through our own ongoing awareness of *whatever* is occurring between us and them. Mindfulness in us is noticeable by others as it flows along its own special way. Then they will *experience* the new us. This is triumph not through domineering, we are not conquerors; but triumph through ability to endure, through patience and nonbelligerency. We let reality teach at its own rhythms.

THE MOUSE

To Master Ko Bong

The mouse eats cat-food, but the cat-bowl is broken. What does
this mean?

When you see the form to be
transparent,
why stay there,
feasting on
Nothing?

GLOSSARY

Adamantine Teaching. Tibetan Buddhism, under its name of Vajrayāna: the vehicle (yāna) which cuts sharply yet is itself undestructible, as a lightning bolt or a diamond (vajra).

anupassanā. The vision (-passanā, Skt.: -paśyanā) which follows along according to what it is seeing (anu-).

arahat, arahan. (Skt.: arhat, arhan. Chinese: lohan, via arahan, alahan, lahan, to lohan). Lit., a worthy one. One who has gained Awakening after hearing the buddhadhamma.

ātman. Self, taken as a constant, reified entity: the ego of egotistic and of "clear ego boundaries".

bāla. Young, not yet fully developed. Said of a sun recently risen, a moon when crescent, grass of tender new blades, as well as of a child, the childish, the puerile, the foolish. In the Indic word the stage of development is in focus.

bālajana. People (jana) who are **bāla** (not yet fully developed).

bodhi. Enlightenment, or awakening. From the verbal root budh/bodh.

bodhisattva. (Pali: bodhisatta.) A being (sattva, Pali: satta) destined for enlightenment (bodhi). Bodhi-sattva is a compound similar to 'the Cheltenham train' as a train whose destination is Cheltenham.

brahmacariyā. (Skt.: brahmacaryā.) The trip (cariyā, Skt.: caryā) toward Brahma. In Sanskrit this has a general meaning of student. In Hinduism it conventionally means one who is following a vow of celibacy. In Buddhism it refers to the endeavours toward enlightenment (lokuttarasīla) and is often translated as The Spiritual Life, in contrast to living a "moral" life which is still tied into karmic fruitions joyful or painful (lokikasīla).

budh/bodh. A verbal root meaning awaken, become conscious or alert, etc.

buddha. One who is awakened. As a proper name, *the* Buddha refers to Siddhattha (Skt.: Siddhārtha) of the Gautama (Pali: Gotama) family or clan within the Sakka (Skt.: Sakya) people, *after* the awakening or enlightenment.

buddhadhamma. The dhamma (Skt.: dharma) or Supporting Way, Teaching, of the Buddha.

burning karma. The processes of experiencing our karma (Pali: kamma, meaning action, from the verbal root kṛ/kar: do, make, act) in which its nature, arising, developing, ending and manifesting in subsequent "fruit" are all gone through consciously. So called out of the heat produced in this process (energy liberated).

dervish, or darvish. One in the Sufi Order begun by Maulana Jalaludin Rumi of Balkh, Khorasan. The well-known practice of whirling incessantly for a period of time derives from the teaching carried on by this Order.

deva. Lit., a shining or bright being. A divine being. The conventional Sanskrit term for a king. From the verbal root div/diu/dy(e)u, as in divine, diurnal, dyeus/Zeus, and meaning shine, lighten up.

dhamma. (Skt.: dharma.) Lit., that which supports, maintains, from the verbal root dhṛ/dhar meaning support, keep, hold, bear, convey, endure, contain. Used referring to that which (a) supports the world in general, as the Way (Tao) of the world; legalised as Natural Law, moralised as Duty. Or, to that which (b) supports the world as an enlightening understanding (Teaching), or as (c) the nature of something, or as (d) the various particular moments within the overall flow of reality, all particulars of consciousness, whence it is said, Sabbe dhammā anattā, All experiences are non-Self.

dharma. See **dhamma, buddhadhamma.**

dukkha. (Skt.: duḥkha.) Pain, discontent, rough times, torment.

gate, gate, pāragate, pārasamgate. From a Buddhist Sanskrit chant, continuing: bodhi svaha (bodhi: awakening, svaha: an exclamation such as Well said, Amen, Oh yes, Quite so). The -gate- form in these words is syntactically either the vocative of gati (O the going) or the locative of gata (in being gone, in being in the state of).

Indic. A branch of the Indo-European Language Family. Its members include Vedic, Classical Sanskrit, Pāli, Māgadhī, Apabramṣa, modern Hindi, Punjābi, Marāthi, Gujarāti, and so on.

Ishq'allah. Part of the Sufi expression ishq'allah ma'abud li'llah, The Totality of Reality is the process of loving, and what is beloved, and what loves. ("God is love, beloved, and lover.")

kalyāṇa. Good, nourishing, inspiring. From a verbal root, kal, meaning impel or push onwards.

kalyāṇa mitta. (Skt.: kalyāṇa mitra.) A good friend, an inspiring friend. A name for the meditation teacher in the vipassanā tradition.

kalyāṇa-mittatā-vimutti-sutta. The talk (discourse, sutta, Skt.: sūtra) on freedom (vimutti, Skt.: vimukti, release, liberation) through good (kalyāṇa) friendship (mittatā, Skt.: mitratā).

karma. See **burning karma**.

Karuṇa-pati. A name meaning lit., Guardian or Lord of Compassion.

Krishna. Lit., The Dark One, the dark-blue-skinned avatar of Vishnu. Krishna knows the senses (Go-vinda), and is the lover of Rādhā and the other cowherdesses.

lokikasīla. A way of acting (sīla) which takes place on the karmic level involving pain and satisfaction, which is, that is, worldly (lokika).

lokuttarasīla. A way of acting (sīla) which is beyond the level of merit/evil, which is beyond the worldly (lokuttara).

mahāsattva. Lit., a great being. A transcendent bodhisattva, that is, one *not* in human form. For more, see Hans Schumann, *Buddhism*, pp. 112f, which gives a more precise account than at either E. Conze, *Buddhist Wisdom Books*, p. 23, or at M. L. Matics, trans., Shantideva's *Entering the Path of Enlightenment*, p. 310.

Mahāyānists. Followers of the Mahāyāna Teachings, the developed thought of the Buddhist Tradition of several centuries after the Buddha (about the beginnings of the Christian Era.) This term is in contrast with Hīnayāna, a derogatory term for earlier ("pristine", "Southern") Buddhism. For more, see H. Schumann, *op. cit.*, pp. 91-94.

Māra. A personification of the tendencies toward unalertness, being deadened to experience. Later taken as a woman (Mārā), Māra was originally a man, the father of the three forms of stupefaction which appeared in the last watch of the night before the Buddha's enlightenment, as Māra's three daughters Ragā (Excited Desire), Aratī (Discontent), and Taṇhā (Skt.: Tṛṣṇā, Thirst, "Grabby" Desire).

Māyā. Lit., an artifice, a deceit, a fraud, trick, or illusion. In Vedānta, unreality as the illusion that there is a reality separate from and other from the Totality, from Deus-sive-Natura, from the Sufic mystical Allah.

Nāga. A hooded serpent. After the Buddha became Awakened, he sat in meditation for 49 days. During this time it began to rain. A nāga wrapped itself around the Buddha and used its hood as an umbrella to shelter the Buddha. The Nāga is sometimes represented as a dragon.

Nāga-Buddha-rūpa. A statue (rūpa, q.v.) of the Buddha with Nāga.

namas-te. Lit., bowing to you. Conventionally a salutation of respect, both Hello and Good-bye, as are Aloha, Shalom, Salaam. In its deeper meaning (paramārtha) it may be glossed 'I honour that within you which is beyond the superficiality of conditioning.'

nirvāṇa. (Pali: nibbāna.) Popularly said to derive from nir+vā, thus meaning "blowing out" (a fire, etc.). This is too active an image. The image of a fire burning itself out when we no longer add fuel to its process is more to the meaning of nirvāṇa. The state free of torment and strife, nirvāṇa is not the same as extinction of life (see **vibhava-taṇhā**). Traditional commentaries such as the *Abhidhammattha Sangaha* analyse it as freedom (nir-) from desire (-vāna). The Buddha described nibbāna or nirvāṇa as the greatest happiness (*Dhammapada*, v. 203).

om. A sound held to represent all sounds. Composed of a-u-m it soundwise embodies reality (since a = Vishnu, u = Shiva, m = Brahma) and so indicates in language all that is beyond language: "all that we may say here is but a pointing to what is beyond these mere words". The sound is held to have physical powers we can experience by constant repetition. (Try and test it out!).

Pali. A Middle-Indic language (see 'Indic'). Used for the preservation of the Theravāda tipiṭaka.

pārami. (Skt.: pāramitā.) Quality brought to full development or "perfection" (its usual translation), traditionally given as six pāramitās (Mahāyāna) or ten pāramis (Theravāda).

pārasaṃgate. See **gate, gate, ...**

rūpa. Form, shape, physical manifestation, image, statue.

sādhu. Success! Well done! Excellent!

saṃsāra. The integrated (saṃ-) on-flowing (-sāra) stream of life. Often translated as The Wheel of Birth and Rebirth.

saṃyutta-nikāya. A nikāya (collection or major unit), the third of five which together compose the sutta-pitaka of the **tipiṭaka**, q.v. It appears in translation under the title *Kindred Sayings*.

sati. Mindfulness, alertness, recollectedness (Skt.: smṛti), from a verbal root smṛ, recall.

sati-paṭṭhāna. (Skt.: smṛty-upasthāna.) The (four) foundations (paṭṭhāna, Skt.: upasthāna) of mindfulness (sati, Skt.: smṛti.)

Shiva. The embodiment (mūrti)—in the Hindu tripartite system (tri-mūrti)—of analysis, destruction, and, later, regeneration. He is also called Naṭa-rāja (Ruler of the Dance).

sīla. (Skt.: śīla, habit, custom, disposition, character, uprightness.) A customary mode of action, word, and thought, either natural (pakati-sīla, Skt.: prakṛti-śīla) or through a discipline of rules (paññatti-sīla, Skt.: prajñapti-śīla). Often translated as Morality.

sutta. (Skt.: sūtra.) A talk or discourse of the Buddha. For more see P. Yampolsky, *The Platform Sutra of the Sixth Patriarch,* p. 125, fn. 1.

tantra. Lit., a means (-tra) for expansion (tan-). That which we use to become less constricted. A practice which carries on through immersion and saturation (a gourmand of life), rather than by control and selectivity. Cf. **yoga.**

Theravāda. The doctrine (-vāda) of the Elders (thera-), preserved in Pali. Also called Pali Buddhism or Southern Buddhism, Sri Lanka having been an early home for this tradition. One among those Schools denegratingly referred to as Hīnayāna. See **Mahayanists.**

tipiṭaka. (Skt.: tripiṭaka.) The three (ti-) baskets or collections (-piṭaka) composing the core of the Theravāda dhamma. Consists of the Vinaya-piṭaka (Procedural and Criminal Law), the Sutta-piṭaka (Discourse Collection), and the Abhidhamma-piṭaka (Abstract Psychology).

U Ba Khin Tradition. A particular form of vipassana meditation in which great emphasis is placed on the practice of concentrative awareness of the body, in mindfulness of breath at the nose and in 'sweeping' one's attention systematically through the body. The school takes its name from the twentieth century Burmese vipassana meditation teacher, U Ba Khin. See further the discussion of 'samathapubbangama-vipassana' under the entry **vipassana meditation.**

vibhava-taṇhā. (Skt.: vibhava-tṛṣṇā.) The thirst (taṇhā, Skt.: tṛṣṇā) for vibhava, for the end (vi-) of ongoing process (bhava), for extinction.

vinaya. See **tipiṭaka.**

vipassanā. (Skt.: vipaśyanā.) Clear (vi-), immediate, intuitive seeing (-passanā, Skt.: paśyanā), free from preconception. Insight into how things are, not how we thought them to be. See also **vipassana meditation.**

vipassana meditation. In the Pali language this is termed vipassanā-bhāvanā. Literally, this bhāvanā of vipassanā is simply the effecting, producing, furthering or cultivation (bhāvanā) of insight (vipassanā). Traditionally, two forms of insight cultivation are mentioned. In one of these, insight is preceded by a concentration of consciousness producing a mental tranquillity or samatha (Buddhist Skt.: śamatha). This is termed vipassanā which has samatha going before it (-pubbaṅgama), or samatha-pubbaṅgama-vipassanā. See here **U Ba Khin Tradition.** In the other of these, the meditator (yogi) does not base the insight cultivated, on a tranquillity practice. The yogi is then called one (-ika) who has as vehicle (yāna) insight (vipassanā) which is pure (suddha, Skt.: śuddha), or a suddha-vipassanā-yānika. Another name for such a yogi is one (-aka) who has bare insight, insight (vipassanā) which is bare, simple, unmixed (with samatha practice), or sukkha (Skt.: śuṣka), meaning literally dry, waterless, 'not watered down'. In Pali this yogi is called a sukkha-vipassaka.

yoga. Lit., a yoking. That by which we discipline ourselves. A practice which carries on by control and selectivity, rather than through immersion and saturation. Cf. **tantra.**

Some available books on Buddhist Vipassanā Meditation and
Psychology, and on Buddhism

The titles of authors (Achaan, Lama, Prince, Rinpoche, Sayadaw, Thera) are given but not used to determine alphabetical ordering.

Buddhaghosa. *The Path of Purification (Visuddhimagga)*. Bhik-
khu Nyāṇamoli (Ñāṇamoli Thera), translator.

Achaan Cha. *A Still Forest Pool: Insight Meditation* (compiled
by Jack Kornfield).

Edward Conze. *Buddhist Wisdom Books.*

The Dhammapada.

Dharmarakṣita. *The Wheel of Sharp Weapons*, with Commentary by Geshe Ngawang Dhargye.

V.R. Dhiravamsa. *The Dynamic Way of Meditation.*

_____. *The Middle Path.*

_____. *New Approach to Buddhism.*

_____. *The Real Way to Awakening.*

_____. *Turning to the Source.*

Mitchell Ginsberg. *The Inner Palace: Mirrors of Psychospirituality in Divine & Sacred Wisdom-Traditions.*

____. *The Orchard of the Outer Courtyard: Psychospirituality
in the World.* MS.

___. *Peace and War and Peace, and Other Poems.* MS.

___. *Calm, Clear, and Loving: Soothing the Distressed Mind,
Healing the Wounded Heart (Reflections on Nietzsche, Ja-
net, Freud; Psychotherapy, Love, and Mindfulness).* MS.

___ & Françoise Ginsberg. *Tango Tantras: The Embrace of
Yearning and Love.* MS.

Daniel Goleman. *The Meditative Mind.*

___. *Emotional Intelligence.*

Joseph Goldstein. *The Experience of Insight.*

Lama Anagarika Govinda. *The Psychological Attitude of Early
Buddhist Philosophy.*

Thich Nhat Hanh. *Transformation & Healing: Sutra on the
Four Establishments of Mindfulness.*

___. *Peace Is Every Step: The Path of Mindfulness in Everyday
Life*

Hongzhi. *Cultivating the Empty Field: The Silent Illumination of Zen Master Hongzhi.*

U Ba Khin. *The Essentials of Buddhadhamma in Meditation Practice.*

Jack Kornfield. *Living Dharma.*

___. *A Path with Heart.*

___. *The Wise Heart.*

Ledi Sayadaw. *Manual of Insight (Vipassanā Dīpanī).*

Mahāsi Sayadaw. *Practical Insight Meditation.*

Lama Mipham. *Calm and Clear.*

Nyanaponika Thera. *The Heart of Buddhist Meditation.*

Walpola Rahula. *What The Buddha Taught.*

___. *Zen and the Taming of the Bull.*

Śantideva [Shantideva]. *Bodhicaryāvatāra*, also entitled *Entering the Path of Enlightenment* and (Tibetan style) *A Guide to the Bodhisattva's Way of Life (Bodhisattvacaryāvatāra)*

Hans W. Schumann. *Buddhism: An Outline of its Teachings and Schools.*

U Silananda. *The Four Foundations of Mindfulness.*

Sogyal Rinpoche. *Dzogchen and Padmasambhava.*

Soma Thera. *The Way of Mindfulness (The Satipaṭṭhāna Sutta and Commentary).*

Anagarika Sujata. *Beginning to See.*

Prince Vajirañānavarorasa. *A Comment on the Third Step of Advantage* (English of the Thai work, *Dhammavicāraṇa*).

Philip Yampolsky. *The Platform Sūtra of the Sixth Patriarch*, also translated as *The Sutra of Hui Neng.*

These texts are available worldwide, as at Motilal Banarsidass (New Delhi), The Pali Text Society (London), Buddhist Publication Society (Kandy, Sri Lanka), Mahamakut Bookstore (opp. Wat Bovoranives, Phra Sumeru Rd., Bangkok), Bodhi Tree Bookstore (West Hollywood CA), Wisdom Publications (Boston), Blackwell's (Oxford).

BUDDHIST MEDITATION CENTRES

At the following centres, various teachers lead meditation workshops and retreats in which there may be significant variation in size of the meditation group, amount of personal contact with the teacher or amount of emphasis placed on ritual, on traditional vow-taking, and on Buddhist doctrine, in the number of hours of formal practice daily, or in the fees charged. In the Glossary, see the entries vipassanā as yoga and as tantra, U Ba Khin Tradition.

BURMA: Thathana Yeiktha, 16 Hermitage Road, Rangoon.

CANADA: (with Bhikshuni Pema Chödrön) Gampo Abbey, Pleasant Bay, Cape Breton, Nova Scotia B0E 2P0.

_____. Tengye Ling, 11 Madison Ave., Toronto, Ontario M5R 2S2.

FRANCE: (with Herb Elsky) Dechen Chöling, Mas Marvent, 87700 St Yrieix sous Aixc (NW of Limoges).

_____. (with Mitchell Ginsberg) J.-P. Aharonian (Assoc. Française de Méditation Vipassana), 1 rue des Alpes, 2600 Valence.

_____. Kagyu Ling, Château de Plaige, La Boulaye, 71320 Toulon-sur-Arroux (SW of Dijon, NW of Mâcon).

_____. Lerab Ling, L'Engayresque, 34650 Roqueredonde (southwest of le Caylar, via les Rives and Romiguères).

GERMANY: (with Dhiravamsa) Haus der Stille, Mühlenweg 20, 21514 Roseburg (east of Hamburg).

INDIA: Samanvaya Ashram, Bodhgaya 824231, Bihar.

_____. Sayaji U Ba Khin Trust, Vipassana International Academy, Dhammagiri, Igatpuri 422403, Maharashtra.

_____. Tushita Retreat Centre, McLeod Ganj, Dharamsala, Dist. Kangra, Himāchal Pradesh 176219.

MALAYSIA: Malaysian Buddhist Meditation Centre, 355 Jalan Mesjid Negeri, 11600 Penang.

NETHERLANDS: Boeddhayana Centrum, Stephensonstraat 13, 2561 XP Den Haag.

_____. Boeddhayana Centrum, Vechtstraat 73, 1079 JV Amsterdam.

SCOTLAND: Kagyu Samyê Ling Tibetan Centre, Eskdalemuir, nr. Langholm, Dumfriesshire.

SPAIN: (with Dhiravamsa) Centro Milarepa, C/ La Naval, 167, 2°, 35008 Las Palmas de Gran Canaria, Isla Gran Canaria.

SRI LANKA: Forest Hermitage, Kandy.

USA (by state):

[CA] Buddha Sāsana Foundation, Attn: Alan Clements, 45 Oak Rd., Larkspur CA 94939.

[CA] (with Ruth Denison) Desert Vipassana Meditation Center, Dhamma Dāna, HC-1, Box 250, Joshua Tree CA 92250.

[CA] Land of Medicine Buddha, 5800 Prescott Rd., Soquel CA 95073.

[CA] (with Jack Kornfield) Spirit Rock Meditation Center, 5000 Sir Francis Drake Blvd., Woodacre CA 94973.

[CA] Thubten Dhargye Ling, 3500 E. 4th Street, Long Beach CA 90814.

[CA] Zen Center of Los Angeles, 923 S. Normandie Ave., Los Angeles CA 90006.

[CO] Thubten Shedrup Ling, 1301 N. Weber St., Colorado Springs CO 80932.

[CO] Wat Buddhavararam, 4801 Julian St., Denver CO 80221.

[FL] Thubten Kunga Ling, 7970 Little Lane, Boca Raton FL 33433.

[IL] Buddhadharma Meditation Center, 8910 State Route 83, Hinsdale IL 60521.

[MA] Insight Meditation Society, 1230 Pleasant St., Barre MA 01005.

[MA] (with Richard Clarke) Living Dharma Center, Box 304, Amherst MA 01004.

[MD] Wat Thai Washington DC, 13440 Layhill Rd., Silver Spring MD 20906.

[NY] Vajiradhammapadip Temple, 75 California Rd., Mount Vernon NY 10552.

[VT] Karmê Chöling, 369 Patneaude Lane, Barnet VT 05821.

[WV] Bhāvanā Society, Route 1, Box 218-3, High View WV 26808.